THE HOLLYWOOD
Wrap

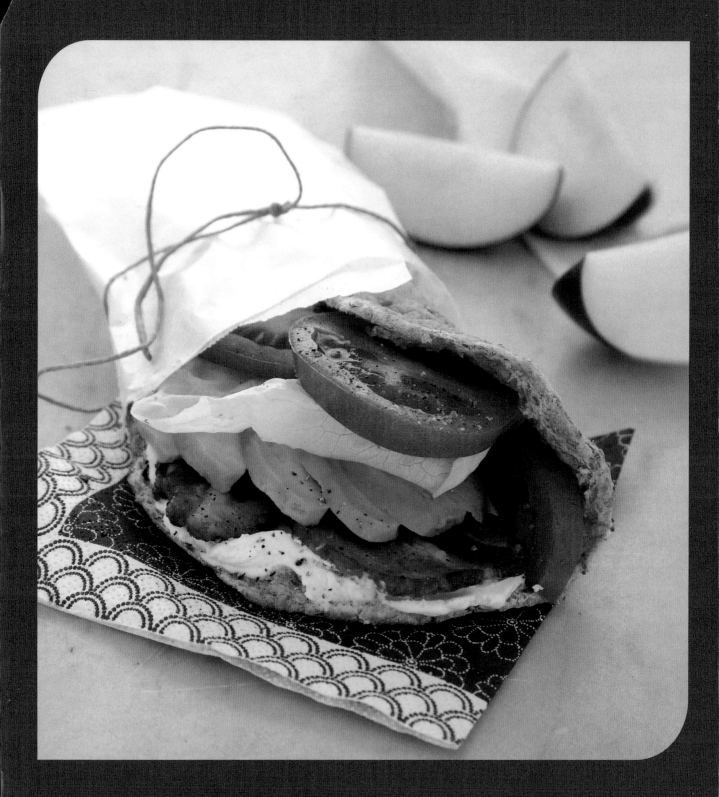

THE HOLLYWOOD
Wrap

★ ★ ★ ★ ★ ★ ★ ★ ★ ★ ★ ★ ★ ★ ★ ★ ★

100 Quick and Easy Meals to Fuel Your Workout
and Help You Lose Weight,
from Celebrity Fitness and Nutrition Expert

Nancy Kennedy

RODALE

© 2011 by Nancy Kennedy

Rodale books may be purchased for business or promotional use or for special sales. For information, please write to:
Special Markets Department, Rodale, Inc., 733 Third Avenue, New York, NY 10017

Printed in the United States of America
Rodale Inc. makes every effort to use acid-free ♾, recycled paper ♻.

Photographs by Heather Weston
Photographs on pages 7 and 178 by David Sobel
Book design by Kara Plikaitis

Library of Congress Cataloging-in-Publication Data

Kennedy, Nancy.
    The Hollywood wrap : 100 quick and easy meals to fuel your workout and help you lose weight, from celebrity fitness and nutrition expert / Nancy Kennedy.
        p.   cm.
    Includes index.
    ISBN 978-1-60529-163-5 paperback
    1. Quick and easy cooking.   2. Low-calorie diet—Recipes.   3. Cookbooks.   I. Title.
    TX833.5.K468   2011
    641.5'63—dc22   2010049487

Distributed to the trade by Macmillan

2 4 6 8 10 9 7 5 3 1   paperback

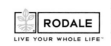

RODALE
LIVE YOUR WHOLE LIFE™

We inspire and enable people to improve their lives and the world around them.
www.rodalebooks.com

To my mom, who always told me I was her little star and could do anything I put my mind to. And to my rock and soul mate, Alex Dmitrevsky, whose vision and support made writing this book possible.

Contents

Foreword

I have spent the last 30 years helping patients achieve and maintain healthy body weights through balanced nutrition and a healthy, active lifestyle.

Obesity-associated diseases now account for a significant portion of total US health expenditures. If we are ever to conquer this growing epidemic, we can't just keep talking about it. We have to do something. Exercise is clearly key, but preparing and eating balanced, nutritious meals to support that healthy, active lifestyle is just as important. However, we all know diets only work when they are followed; ensuring your daily menus contain variety and are fun to eat makes it much more likely that you will stick to your weight-loss goals. And that's where Nancy and her handy meals-in-a-wrap come in.

Like many food trends, the wrap has taken off in California and especially in Hollywood because it is convenient, portable, and endlessly variable. However, when it comes to wraps, don't forget that what's on the outside is as important as what's on the inside. Making wraps with healthy ingredients—from the wrap itself to the nutrient-packed filling within—is what this book is all about.

I have known Nancy as the "Trainer to the Stars" long before that term became fashionable and overused, and for many years she has been the one I turn to when I have a client who needs the right combination of inspiration, sound fitness advice, and nutritional guidance. She has helped many of my clients, including celebrities, politicians, and captains of industry, achieve their weight-loss goals, and if you follow her advice, she will help you, too.

With the current flood of fad diets and celebrity weight-loss memoirs on the shelves today, it is refreshing to find a book based on sound nutrition. Nancy has done a masterful job of creating great-tasting recipes that are also nutritionally balanced and healthful. One excuse my clients often give for consuming fast foods is that there is not enough time within their stressful lives to do things right. With this collection of easy, fast, and fun wrap recipes, that excuse is no longer valid.

David Heber, MD, PhD*
Director, UCLA Center for Human Nutrition
David Geffen School of Medicine
Los Angeles, California

* Dr. Heber's name and title are for identification purposes only. The University of California does not endorse specific products or services as a matter of policy.

Introduction

Why do Hollywood's major stars always look great in movies and music videos, walking down the red carpet at international openings, and sitting through grueling publicity tours?

Because looking good and being in shape are essential to their work and lives. Preparing for a role doesn't just mean learning lines and going to costume fittings. It also includes everything from gaining or losing weight for a particular character to being trim and fit so the camera doesn't add 10 to 20 pounds.

Stars take this responsibility seriously. Very seriously. I know because I'm a personal trainer, nutrition expert, and healthy cook who works with A-list clients such as Halle Berry, Jennifer Lopez, Kevin Costner, Julia Roberts, Shakira, Jessica Biel, and many others, in order to whip them into shape.

I got my start cooking for the stars when I was hired to work with Julia Roberts on location in Chicago for the movie *I Love Trouble.* I emptied out the minibar in Julia's hotel suite, removed room service menus, and brought in a big fridge stocked with fruit and snacks and a blender for protein shakes. When shooting moved to Madison, Wisconsin, I went, too. I cooked at Julia's fully stocked rental home, preparing grilled chicken breasts and vegetables, stuffed baked potatoes, protein shakes, and salads to keep her energy levels up and her weight down. Three meals and snacks a day had to be low in calories, yet tasty and filling.

In Wisconsin, it was easy to cook with ingredients and equipment at my fingertips. But as I began to train and cook for other actors on movie and music video sets where kitchens weren't available, I had to come up with on-the-go, balanced meals. Wraps were the answer! Movie stars on set could eat something quick, healthy, and balanced, without compromising one food group over another.

My wraps contain lean protein, complex carbohydrates, and essential fats that keep my clients looking and feeling great. They're gourmet fast foods that are healthy and have star-level taste.

The Hollywood Wrap features the same easy recipes I make for Hollywood's top stars, movers, and shakers. Each wrap is a complete meal for breakfast, lunch, or dinner. My wraps taste great and help keep off the pounds. Sure, you say, celebs have trainers and nutritionists. That's true, but they are human and still have to do the workouts and eat properly. The most important thing is, you may not be a movie star (yet), but now you can eat and lose weight like one!

Thanks so much for inviting me on your journey to health and wellness. I hope you have as much fun reading the information here as I did writing it for you. I look forward to working with you again soon! Until then, remember to set daily goals for fitness and nutrition, and to not beat yourself up if you have a slip or two along the way. There's always tomorrow!

Best,

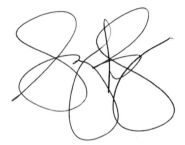

Nancy F. Kennedy

★ The Skinny on Important Nutrients

PROTEIN, COMPLEX CARBOHYDRATES, AND ESSENTIAL FATS

It's amazing how many fad diets there are. All carbs. No carbs. Low fat. No fat. All protein. No protein. Yet none of them deliver on their promise—permanent weight loss.

When it comes to nutrition and food, I believe in balance. There's a reason for every nutrient, so why eliminate one? If someone suggests that you should eliminate one entire food group—be it carbs, protein, or fat—don't listen. Protein is essential for building lean muscle. Don't eliminate carbohydrates. Your body needs complex carbs for energy and fiber. Certain fats are required for healthy hair, skin, and nails. The trick is to eat enough of each group each day to keep your body balanced and working at its full potential. If your breakfast wrap doesn't have enough carbs, have a wrap with some brown rice or quinoa for lunch. Balance is key to everything in life. Remember, eat right, not hype!

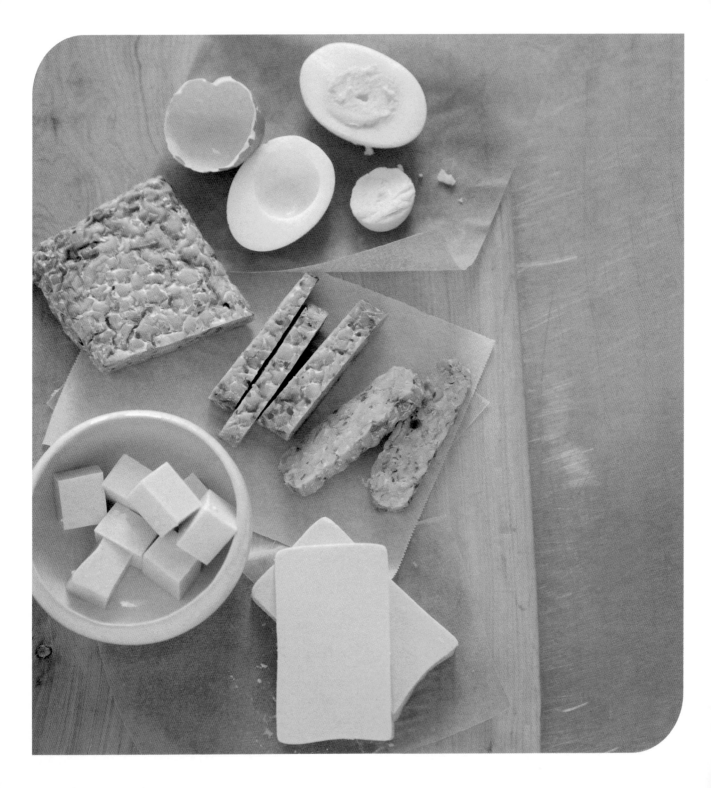

PROTEIN

All tissues, bones, and nerves are made primarily of protein. It's necessary for optimal health, vitality, growth, and development. Proteins are the building blocks for muscles, blood, skin, hair, nails, and internal organs such as the brain and heart. Proteins are vital to many bodily processes, including metabolism, immune function, transport of nutrients, skin integrity, and body tissue growth and repair. Eat proteins that are lean and low in saturated fat such as chicken or turkey breast, canned tuna, top sirloin or filet mignon, and tofu. Add a scoop of protein powder to smoothies or shakes. If you're a vegetarian or vegan, get your protein from nuts, seeds, beans, legumes, and soy products.

MY TOP PROTEIN PICKS

* Chicken: boneless, skinless breasts

* Beef: lean top sirloin and filet

* Turkey: skinless breast or extra-lean ground breast

* Eggs: whole eggs combined with egg whites (one yolk for every three whites)

* Shellfish: crabmeat, shrimp, and lobster

* Fish: flounder, cod, halibut, tuna, and salmon

* Protein powders: low-sugar whey or soy protein powder

* Cheese: fat-free cottage cheese or fat-free ricotta cheese

* Pork: tenderloin

* Tofu: extra-firm

* Tempeh

* Tuna: canned solid white, packed in water, no salt added

COMPLEX CARBOHYDRATES: BEANS, WHOLE GRAINS AND CEREALS, FRUITS, AND VEGETABLES

Many people are confused when it comes to carbohydrates. Carbohydrates are the body's preferred source of energy, and they provide crucial vitamins, minerals, and nutrients to our diet. What's important is the *type* of carbs you eat. Focus on complex carbs—vegetables, fruit, and whole grains.

Processed foods made from refined carbs whose essential nutrients have been removed (white flour, white rice, and white sugar) tend to be calorie-dense and easy to overeat. Avoid these foods—white bread, cookies, chips, baked desserts, snack foods, etc.—whenever possible. Instead, choose foods made from complex carbohydrates and whole grains, which have most or all of their fiber and nutrients intact.

MY TOP COMPLEX-CARBOHYDRATE PICKS

* Fresh fruit

* Dried beans and other legumes, such as lentils

* Cruciferous vegetables: broccoli, Brussels sprouts, cabbage, cauliflower, kale, bok choy

* Whole grain, high-fiber breads (such as Ezekiel bread)

* Corn, fresh or frozen

* Corn tortillas

* Cereals: Fiber One or All-Bran Complete

* Sweet potatoes

* Whole grain sides: barley, brown rice, bulgur, oatmeal, and quinoa

* Whole wheat tortillas and crackers

* High-protein, whole wheat pasta

* Winter squash: butternut, acorn, and kabocha

ESSENTIAL FATS

Like carbohydrates, fat is an essential nutrient, and no diet should be entirely free of fat. However, successful dieting requires eating "good" rather than "bad" fats. Eat unsaturated fats found in roasted unsalted nuts (cashews and almonds), seeds (sunflower and pumpkin), and avocados for the nutrients that support hair, nail, and skin growth. The right fats provide energy for our muscles (including our hearts), support cell walls, and enable the body to circulate, store, and absorb the fat-soluble vitamins A, D, E, and K. Fat protects our vital organs, provides insulation against extreme heat and cold, supplies us with the essential fatty acids, like linoleic acid, that our bodies can't make, and makes food taste better by providing extra flavor, texture, and aroma.

Olive oil, preferably the extra-virgin variety, is another healthy fat you can incorporate into your meals. Olive oil contains substances called polyphenols, which widen blood vessels and lower blood pressure. It increases metabolic rate and helps people control their weight.

Eliminating all fat from your diet can make food inedible, and it is really not recommended. There are ways to reduce the amount you consume without sacrificing flavor. Fruit puree is a good substitute for butter in baked goods; use nonfat plain yogurt in dressings; and moisten turkey meatballs with low-fat, low-sodium chicken broth.

Research shows that by eating more omega-3 fats, especially the kind found in fish, you can fight heart disease and lose weight. Omega-3s relax constricted arteries, heal artery walls, and stabilize heart cells to maintain regular rhythm. They have been shown to block production of hormone-like compounds that contribute to joint inflammation and even to fight depression. Best sources? Salmon, fresh tuna, and trout, preferably the wild-caught variety.

MY TOP ESSENTIAL-FAT PICKS

* ★ Avocado

* ★ Salmon, tuna, and trout

* ★ Flax meal

* ★ Nuts, soy nuts, and seeds, unsalted

* ★ Nut butters, unsalted, no sugar

* ★ Extra-virgin olive oil

HOW TO USE HOLLYWOOD WRAPS TO ACHIEVE YOUR WEIGHT-LOSS GOALS

My wraps are a boon to dieters because they are a convenient and easy way to control portion size and caloric intake. Best of all, they add fun and variety to your diet. Too often people trying to lose weight eat the same foods every day: oatmeal for breakfast, a big salad for lunch, and grilled fish and vegetables for dinner. Sound familiar? The upside is that it's predictable and safe; the downside is that it's boring. Boredom is one of the main factors that lead to unhealthy food choices. When you don't look forward to your meals, you're more tempted to snack or blow off your meals entirely in

favor of something truly unhealthy. And when that happens, your weight-loss program flies out the window. (The same holds true for your fitness program, which is why I recommend switching up your exercise routine every few weeks. See page 12.) Fortunately, you could have a Hollywood Wrap for every breakfast, lunch, and dinner for a week without repeating a single one—plus a few snacks to boot!

If, on the other hand, you are someone who relies on meal replacements like protein shakes or fitness bars, you'll find substituting a wrap instead will leave you fuller and more satisfied, and provide more balanced nutrition than those pre-fab options.

Most importantly, having a wrap in your office fridge or made up and ready to take along as you head out the door in the morning is your insurance policy against those truly bad food choices we all make when we're rushed, stressed, and starving! Start your day with a hearty breakfast wrap and you derail the temptation to order a muffin along with your morning joe. Bring a wrap for lunch and you'll skip the burger-and-fries or "healthy" salad (that's actually drenched in fatty dressing and topped with caloric diet busters like cheese, croutons, and candied nuts). Feel free to keep right on wrapping and rolling through dinner, or simply eat a sensibly portioned meal to end your day (and lay off the alcohol, especially if you're looking to drop a significant number of pounds).

I recommend that my clients eat a wrap for at least one meal each day, usually breakfast or lunch, so that they start the day fueled with something nutritious and calorie-controlled.

I also suggest that my clients reduce their consumption of meat and choose a vegetarian or vegan wrap one or two days a week—or even for one meal each day.

A word about portion size in this book. One serving for the recipes counts as a single, all-in-one meal portion, and, with very few exceptions, clocks in at 250 to 400 calories for a full wrap. So if you choose your wraps with care (as we have in the meal plans that follow), you could actually eat a full wrap for breakfast, lunch, and dinner with two sensible snacks and still not exceed 1,200 calories per day (a good target for those looking to reduce their weight at a steady, healthy pace).

However, you should feel free to cut the wraps into halves or thirds if smaller, more frequent meals help keep you feeling full and satisfied. I rarely eat more than a half of a wrap at a time, and sometimes I even divide them into thirds or quarters and simply graze throughout the day. My Granola Energy Wrap (page 29), for example, is full of good complex carbs and protein, but it's also high in calories; I recommend you cut it into quarters and enjoy it over the course of a day or two. As long as the total calories don't exceed your target, you'll be getting great nutrition and eating reasonably. And how much healthier is it to treat yourself to a half of a Power Fruit Wrap (page 26) than to hit up the vending machine? You'll have a

much easier time making it through the day with something substantial and slow-digesting in your stomach. The key is to stay hungry (but not starving!) and keep your metabolism revved up and burning calories all day while sustaining your energy.

Portion size should also reflect your activity level and gender. If you exercise 4 or 5 days a week (and I'm not talking about 10 minutes of light aerobics a day), you are considered an athlete and require a higher caloric intake. For example, when I was working with Jessica Biel and Ryan Reynolds for *Blade: Trinity,* Ryan, who is 6 foot 4, required a minimum of 4 whole albacore tuna wraps a day—in addition to all the greens, vegetables, and protein drinks he could consume. Jessica required a similar eating regimen and ate a whole albacore tuna wrap at each meal. For a less active lifestyle, you may find that just half of a very protein-dense wrap does the trick and quells your hunger. Just try to keep an eye on total calories and grams of protein per day. Your protein intake should be about 0.36 grams of protein per pound of body weight, which is about 47 grams per day for a 130-pound person, or between 0.5 and 0.7 per pound of body weight for a very active person (that's about 140 grams for a 200-pound athlete).

For more substantial meals, know that you can always accompany wraps with a big green salad tossed with any of the low-fat dressings in this book or some in-season green vegetables. And don't forget that many of the wrap fillings can be served on a bed of salad greens, high-protein, whole wheat pasta, or steamed vegetables. Think outside the wrap!

MEAL PLANS

The two meal plans that follow will show you how to incorporate Hollywood Wraps into your daily routine, whether you are actively trying to shed weight or you simply want to maintain the healthy weight you are now. Feel free to mix it up as you like; these are simply guidelines for getting a varied, balanced mix of flavors and nutrients throughout the day and week.

However, don't feel that you have to start from scratch every single day. It's efficient and smart to prepare multiple wraps at a time and eat them throughout the week. For example, you could make the Frittata of Champions Wraps (page 30) and have one for breakfast on Monday, one for lunch on Tuesday, and another for breakfast on Wednesday (or half of a wrap for a morning and afternoon snack). A Philly Cheese Steak Wrap (page 168) can be lunch on Thursday, dinner on Friday, and a snack on Saturday (minus the tortilla). That way you'll get plenty of variety in your menus without having to prepare an array of new meals each day. Be sure to label your wraps so you can just grab and go, and eat them within a day or two of preparing them. Precook your pro-

teins (e.g., chicken breasts, lean beef) and freeze them so they are ready to pop into a recipe at a moment's notice. The whole point is to eat clean and lean, using all-natural proteins, fruits, and vegetables, and favoring complex carbs and essential fats. Be creative, have fun, and stay active, and your body will reward you.

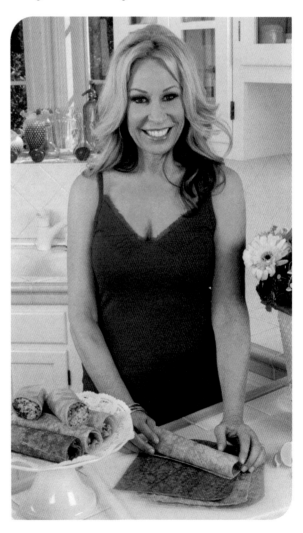

WEIGHT-LOSS PLAN

Low in calories, yet filling and flavorful, these menus—and 6 days of exercise—will help you drop a few pounds in a short amount of time.

Monday

Breakfast: Egg-white omelet with spinach, tomatoes, and fat-free Cheddar

Snack: 2 links Jennie-O turkey sausage

Lunch: 1 **Tuna Melt** (page 159)

Snack: 1 cup steamed edamame

Dinner: 1 **Veggie Burger Wrap** (page 7)

Tuesday

Breakfast: 1 **Scrambled Tofu and Eggs with Salsa Wrap** (page 38)

Snack: 1 cup 0% plain Greek yogurt with $\frac{1}{4}$ cup berries

Lunch: 1 **Butternut Squash Enchilada** (page 57)

Snack: 1 cup low-fat trail mix

Dinner: 2 **Turkey Breast Meatballs with Fat-Free Marinara Sauce** (page 135), $\frac{1}{2}$ cup cooked brown rice, 2 tablespoons fresh salsa

Wednesday

Breakfast: $\frac{1}{2}$ **Power Fruit Wrap** (page 26)

Snack: 2 thin slices turkey breast with mustard

Lunch: 1 **AB&J** (page 49)

Snack: 100-calorie snack pack of whole wheat crackers

Dinner: Grilled salmon with mustard-dill sauce, steamed asparagus with lemon juice

Thursday

Breakfast: 1 **Bacon, Egg, and Cheese Wrap** (page 36)

Snack: 1 cup red peppers, $\frac{1}{4}$ cup roasted unsalted almonds

Lunch: Sashimi over greens with miso dressing

Snack: 1 apple with 1 tablespoon almond butter

Dinner: 1 **Sautéed Portobello Wrap** (page 84)

Friday

Breakfast: 1 cup 0% plain Greek yogurt with $\frac{1}{2}$ cup berries

Snack: 2 **Minced Chicken Lettuce Wraps** (page 123)

Lunch: Greek salad with dressing on the side

Snack: 2 **Minced Chicken Lettuce Wraps** (page 123)

Dinner: Baked cod, steamed spinach, tomato-cucumber salad

Saturday

Breakfast: 1 cup oatmeal with ¼ cup berries, skim milk, and 1 teaspoon whey protein (optional)

Snack: 1 cup unsalted whole wheat pretzels

Lunch: 1 **Mu Shu Beef Wrap** (page 164) and **2 Summer Rolls** (page 72)

Snack: 1 cup steamed broccoli, cauliflower, and carrots with fat-free dressing

Dinner: Broiled chicken breast sprinkled with balsamic vinegar and fat-free mozzarella, ½ cup sautéed green beans

Sunday

Breakfast: 1 **Southwestern Scramble Wrap** (page 32)

Snack: 1 cup grapes

Lunch: 1 **Buffalo Tempeh Wrap with Blue Cheese Dressing** (page 54)

Snack: ¼ cup unsalted sunflower seeds

Dinner: High-protein, whole wheat pasta with fat-free **Marinara Sauce** (page 53) and green salad

MAINTENANCE PLAN

You've done it! You stuck to your food plan and worked and sweated off those calories. That bikini is going to look great when you hit the beach in a week! Eating these wraps will keep your weight steady and your body rockin'.

Monday

Breakfast: 1 **Frittata of Champions Wrap** (page 30)

Snack: ½ cup 0% plain Greek yogurt with ¼ cup berries

Lunch: 1 **Chicken-Cashew Salad Wrap** (page 101)

Snack: 2 cups air-popped popcorn

Dinner: Turkey breast meat loaf, steamed broccoli

Tuesday

Breakfast: 1 cup oatmeal with ⅓ cup banana, soy milk, and 1 teaspoon whey protein (optional)

Snack: ½ **Granola Energy Wrap** (page 29)

Lunch: 1 bowl low-sodium broth, 1 small salad with side of fat-free dressing

Snack: 1 apple with 1 tablespoon almond butter

Dinner: 1 **Asian Steak Salad Wrap** (page 166)

Wednesday

Breakfast: ½ **Granola Energy Wrap** (page 29)

Snack: ¼ cup unsalted almonds

Lunch: 1 Grilled Chicken Wrap with Honey-Mustard-Dill Sauce (page 114)

Snack: 1 sliced plum tomato, 1/2 cup fat-free cottage cheese

Dinner: Roasted pork loin, 1 small roasted sweet potato, steamed spinach

Thursday

Breakfast: 1 Kick Start Egg and Sausage Wrap (page 35)

Snack: 1/2 cup cooked chickpeas with fat-free vinaigrette

Lunch: 1 Philly Cheese Steak Wrap (page 168), diced tomatoes (optional)

Snack: 1/2 banana with nut butter

Dinner: Baked chicken and rice, steamed green beans with garlic

Friday

Breakfast: Egg-white omelet with spinach, tomatoes, and fat-free cottage cheese

Snack: 1 cup carrot sticks, 1 ounce fat-free cheese

Lunch: 1 Red Pepper, Mushroom, and Goat Cheese Wrap (page 44)

Snack: 1/2 cup steamed edamame sprinkled with sesame seeds

Dinner: 1 Lamb-Couscous Wrap (page 170)

Saturday

Breakfast: 1 whole grain bagel, scooped out and spread with a smear of nut butter and fruit spread

Snack: 1 cup 0% plain Greek yogurt

Lunch: 1 Turkey-Swiss Deli Wrap (page 132)

Snack: 1/2 cup low-sugar, fat-free fruit sorbet with 1/2 cup blueberries

Dinner: 1/2 Crab, Shrimp, and Avocado Roll (page 146)

Sunday

Breakfast: 1 Smoking Salmon Wrap (page 40)

Snack: Low-calorie granola bar

Lunch: Mixed green salad with 6 ounces grilled chicken breast and fat-free dressing

Snack: 1 Spinach Pizza Pie Roll (page 52)

Dinner: 1 Crunchie Munchie Tuna Wrap (page 155)

★

The Hollywood Wrap

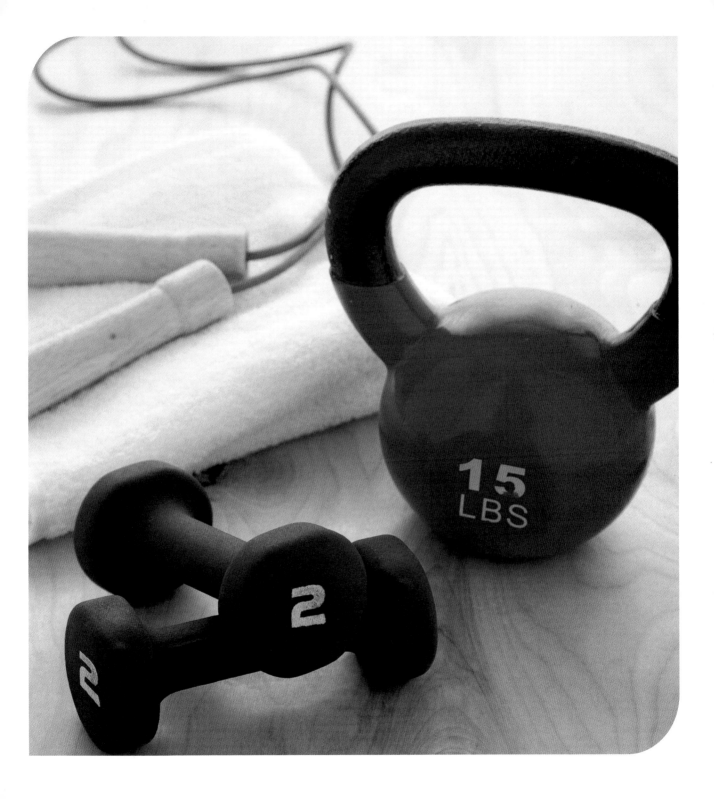

WORK OUT YOUR BODY AND YOUR BRAIN!

Exercise is essential for weight loss, strength, and longevity, as well as for physical and mental health. Scientific studies have long proven the correlation between a healthy mind and a fit body. By using *The Hollywood Wrap,* you're getting a "two-fer." You're going to discover how to improve your body with the knowledge in these pages, and you're going to implement that knowledge to make you super-scintillating, like a Hollywood movie star! Gee, you're going to be smart and gorgeous, too! Look out, Hollywood!

Getting into and staying in shape requires dedication and planning—it doesn't just happen. Ask any actor or movie star. They work hard at staying healthy, fit, and trim. You can do the same. Stay focused and be prepared. Start the day with an intense, effective workout. Shop for and plan your meals ahead of time so you always know what you're going to eat for breakfast, lunch, and dinner for as much as a week at a time. This way, if you fill your fridge with Hollywood Wraps, you won't give in and eat foods that derail you from your goals.

A realistic first goal might be to take a brisk walk, lift weights, jump rope, go to yoga or Pilates class, or ride a bike. Set a goal of 6 days a week to do at least 30 minutes of exercise a day to start. If you miss a day of exercise or slip on your diet a bit, it's okay.

Just wake up the next morning determined to pick yourself up, dust yourself off, and start over. There's no such thing as a bad workout. Remember, this lifestyle is for you and only you. Do the best workout you can do, 6 days a week! Besides dieting jump starts, workouts have so many more benefits beyond a flat tummy or toned biceps. You'll sleep better. You'll feel energized. You'll be more focused at home and at work. You'll be happier! You'll be living the Hollywood Wrap lifestyle just like the movie stars!

WATER ROCKS!

Why do movie stars have such great skin? Because they drink water. Plenty and plenty of water. (Paparazzi who take candid photos of stars know they are *always* carrying water bottles!)

Your body requires water to hydrate your muscles and spread nutrients throughout your system. The energy-burning process of metabolism needs water to work effectively. Lack of water, like a lack of food, can impair your body's metabolic rate.

If the tap water where you live isn't tasty or is filled with chemicals, purchase a 2-quart pitcher with a water filter. Try to drink two pitchers over the course of each day. Add some orange, lemon, lime, or cucumber slices to add flavor. Herbs such as mint or lemon verbena are delicious, too.

★ Wrappers for Your Wraps

The actual wrapper for your wrap does more than contain the filling. It provides visual appeal, flavor, and nutrition.

When wraps first came on the scene, white flour tortillas were the standard option, which gave tortillas a bad "wrap" nutritionally. White flour is processed to remove the bran and germ, mainly to improve its shelf life, but this also strips it of valuable nutrients and fiber, making white flour tortillas high in calories and low in nutritional value and fiber content. Fortunately, as more and more consumers demanded healthful food options, whole grain tortillas and other flatbread products became available. Whole grain flours include the grain's nutritious bran, germ, and endosperm. Breads and tortillas made from whole grains are considered complex carbohydrates. Their nutrients are digested slowly and keep you feeling full, a benefit you don't get from simple carbohydrates.

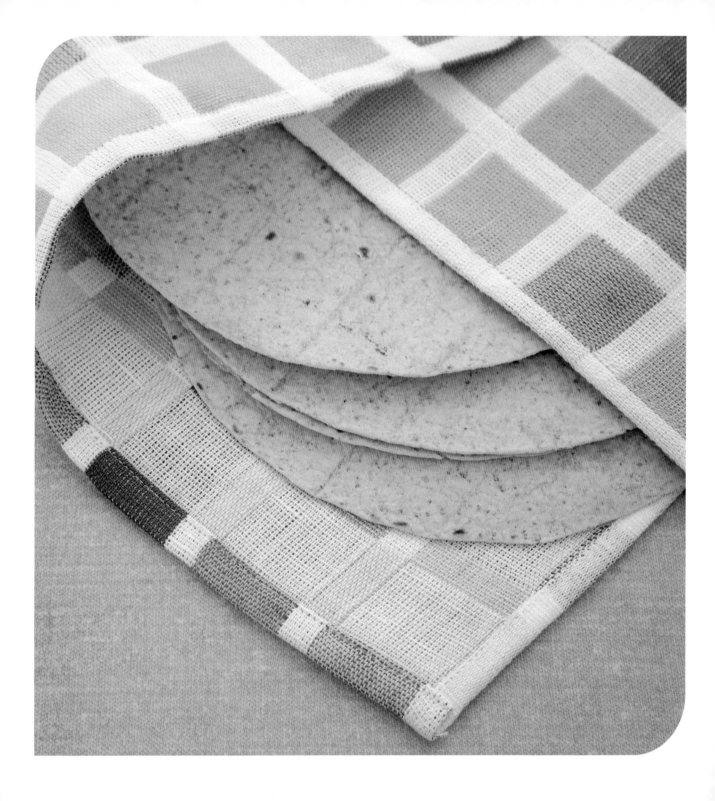

So, there are good reasons to choose your wrappers with care. There are several things you should consider when reading a food label, starting with the serving size on the package. How many servings are included? Most tortillas and pitas are considered one serving, but don't assume that's the case; if the label says each represents two servings, then you must multiply all the amounts by two. (This is equally true for many other food products, particularly highly caloric snack foods and drinks.)

Calorie content is also important when considering a wrap. Compare different brands and become familiar with the labels. Some wraps get most of their calories from saturated fats or trans fats; these are the brands that you don't want to buy. Instead, choose brands that derive most of their calories from proteins and good carbohydrates. These are *good* calories, unlike the calories you get from saturated fats. Saturated fats are the artery-clogging fats that contribute to heart disease and diabetes. There should be zero or very minimal saturated fats in your wraps. Also, look out for trans fats. These cheap, solid fats are being taken off the market as science discovers how detrimental they are to our health.

The wraps you purchase should also be cholesterol free. Check the nutrition label. High cholesterol levels can lead to heart disease over time. Cholesterol creates plaque in your arteries, which decreases circulation and impairs the health of your heart, brain, and limbs. People who have poor circulation tend to have low energy levels, failing memories, decreased visual acuity, and various aches and pains. You can prevent plaque buildup in your arteries by healthy eating and exercising 6 days per week. You have to be persistent though, because lowering cholesterol takes months. So keep encouraging yourself to stay on track each and every day!

Check the sodium content in each wrap. Some can have as much as 10 percent or more of your daily intake of salt. The less salt you eat, the less water you retain and the less you weigh. A high-sodium diet can lead to high blood pressure and heart disease. The wraps in this book are very low in salt, somewhere below the 10 percent mark of the daily allowable intake. This rule of thumb helps keep the total amount of sodium I consume below the 100 percent point as I head toward the end of my day. Making seemingly small choices, like choosing a low-sodium wrap over a salty one, add up to significant dietary changes.

Purchase high-fiber wraps, those with the highest number of fiber grams per serving you can find. Fiber is important in our diets when it comes to preventing intestinal diseases like diverticulitis and colon cancer, and it helps you feel fuller longer. Contrary to popular belief, fiber supplements are a less effective way to improve your fiber intake than simply eating food rich in soluble and insoluble fiber, like bran, whole grains, vegetables, and fruit, as well as beans, peas, and oats. Soluble fiber dissolves in water and keeps you feeling full. It also helps reduce the risk for diabetes and lowers your cholesterol. Insoluble fiber keeps the digestive system running regularly. Our bodies need both in order to keep our energy up, our blood sugar and cholesterol down, and our digestive system healthy.

Here are some of my favorite wrappers. You'll find many of them in supermarkets and even more at natural food stores. New products are coming onto the market every day. Although I offer specific wrap suggestions in each recipe, feel free to use whatever you have on hand, or substitute lettuce leaves for a tortilla. Keep all tortillas refrigerated in airtight packages, and keep an eye on the use-by date on the package.

Flour tortillas: Whole wheat tortillas made without lard are the wraps I use most often and are nutritionally superior to white flour or corn tortillas. They come in a range of sizes, from 5 inches to almost a foot in diameter. Remember, the larger the tortilla, the more calories it is likely to contain. I stick to 8-inch tortillas to control portion size effectively.

My favorite tortillas are made by a company called Tumaro's. I use them in my commercial food line and at home because they meet all my nutrition requirements and come in a variety of flavors. If your market doesn't carry them, or doesn't carry the full range of flavors, ask the store manager to order them. (Visit www.tumaros.com for additional information.)

I also use a brand of tortillas called Nopaltilla. They're just $5\frac{1}{2}$ inches in diameter, but they pack a nutritional wallop because they're made with nopales (the fleshy leaves of the prickly pear cactus) and mixed with stone-ground whole corn kernels. A serving of two tortillas contains just 100 calories, no sodium, 2 percent fat (none from saturated fats, trans fats, or cholesterol), 10 percent daily calcium allowance, 4 percent daily iron allowance, 12 percent daily fiber allowance, no sugar, and 8 percent carbs. And they're organic. They are 100 percent natural and contain no preservatives. Heat and store them as you would other tortillas.

Flavored tortillas: Many markets carry tortillas with green spinach, red tomato, black beans, and the like added to the dough and flavored with spices or herbs. These colorful tortillas are usually white flour–based, and those attractive additives usually don't significantly improve their low nutritional profile. Some flavored whole grain tortillas are now available to the food service industry, so it probably won't be long before home cooks can buy them at natural food markets. For the time being, though, whole wheat tortillas are your best choice.

Multigrain tortillas: These are made from a mixture of flours and other grain products, such as bran, which add bulk while they lower the total carbohydrates. This entitles some companies to label their brands "low carb."

Gluten-free varieties: It's much easier to find gluten-free tortillas—such as those made from millet, teff, brown rice, and flax meal—in the markets these days, which, of course, is good news for people who can't tolerate gluten, but these can also add variety to anyone's wraps. Those who are gluten intolerant should know that wraps made with spelt and sprouted wheat are not gluten free.

Corn tortillas: Some people love corn tortillas best of all. I only love them when they're fresh, right off the tortilla maker, purchased at my local Latin market. If you can't bear to live without them, here is how to refresh and soften them. If you have a gas stove, set the corn tortilla right on the burner grill over medium heat and let the flames tickle the tortilla for 30 seconds or so. Using tongs, flip the tortilla to the other side and let the flames lightly char the other side. This helps the tortillas become flexible and is an excellent way to revive otherwise rubbery corn tortillas. You can also heat them in the microwave for a few seconds to soften them, though I'm not keen on the appliance.

Rice papers: Available at Asian markets and in the ethnic food aisle of many supermarkets, rice paper wrappers are made from only rice, water, and salt. These translucent white rounds are used to make Vietnamese summer rolls, which are filled with shrimp, thin rice or bean (cellophane) noodles, and herbs, and accompanied by a dipping sauce. They can be put into service with other fillings, as

Spice (or Herb) Up Your Wrappers

It is easy to add a bit of color and flavor to plain whole wheat tortillas. Heat a nonstick skillet over medium heat. Place a tortilla in the skillet and heat without flipping it, until the tortilla is warm and pliable, about 1 minute. Lightly brush the unheated side with water to barely moisten the surface. (You can also spray the tortilla with olive or canola oil from a non-aerosol oil mister—which can be purchased at kitchenware stores—for another layer of flavor.) Sprinkle the moistened area with the dried herbs or ground spices of your choice. Dried herbs, such as thyme, basil, or oregano, have the best visual appeal and flavor. It's best to used dried herbs (but not powdery ground herbs), because chopped fresh herbs tend to fall off the tortilla unless very finely minced. Spice options include ground cinnamon, turmeric, and pure ground chiles, or use spice mixtures (chili powder, curry, Chinese five-spice powder, and Moroccan or Cajun spice blends come to mind). Flip the tortilla and cook just until the underside has dried and the coating adheres without toasting or browning, about 15 seconds.

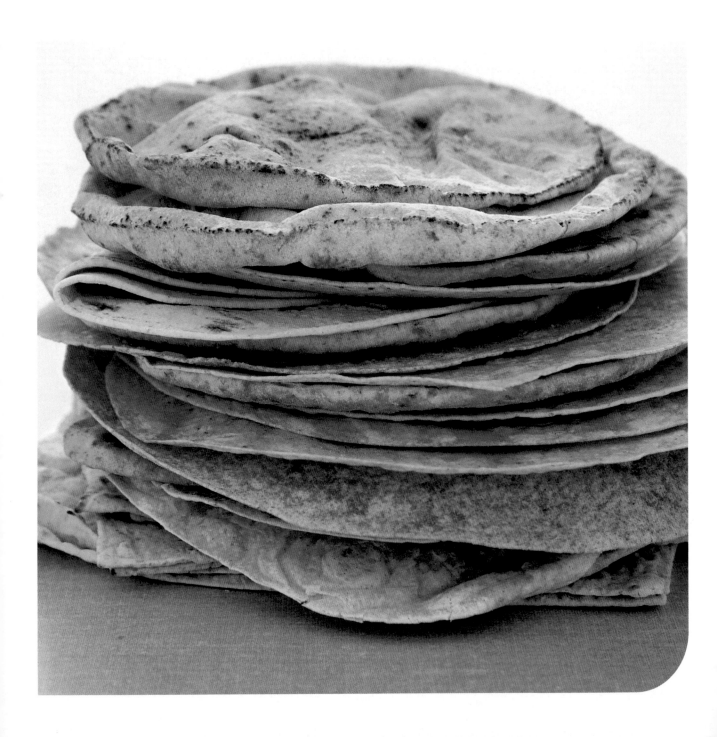

well. They are not whole grain, but are low in calories (just 20 in each one) and fat free. As an occasional change from tortillas they can be part of a healthy diet. Plus, they are very tasty and elegant looking when prepared artistically. Want to impress your friends? Tie translucent rice papers with a little strip of scallion greens.

Rice paper wrappers must be soaked briefly in water to make them pliable before they are filled and folded. Set yourself up with a shallow dish of water and a clean kitchen towel next to the bowl, and have all the fillings ready to go. Slide one wrapper into the water to immerse it and let stand until just softened, 5 to 15 seconds. Remove the rice paper from the water, put it on the towel, and let it sit for 20 to 30 seconds to soak up excess water and make it a bit more pliable. Fill the rice paper and fold as you would a burrito, tucking in the ends as you roll. Rice paper rolls are best when freshly softened, but they can be prepared several hours ahead. Cover them with damp paper towels and plastic wrap, and refrigerate until ready to serve.

Two widely available brands of rice paper wrappers are Red Rose and Three Ladies. Stored airtight at room temperature, they keep for up to a year.

Soy wrappers: Originally used by sushi chefs as an alternative to nori (the pressed seaweed sheets that enclose many sushi rolls), soy wrappers are a new addition to the wrap scene. They are made of soy flour and come in a rainbow of naturally derived colors, including pink, green, and yellow. You'll find soy wrappers at well-stocked Japanese markets and at many online grocers. Store them at room temperature for up to 6 months. Soy wrappers don't require any soaking and are used directly from the package.

Flatbreads: Many ethnic flatbreads, from pita breads to lavash and naan, are now sold in whole wheat versions and make perfect wrappers. You probably won't have to travel far to find them, as they are increasingly carried at supermarkets. **Pita bread** can have a pocket or not. If your pita is too thick to roll up, split it horizontally with a serrated knife. **Naan,** a deliciously chewy Indian flatbread, is similar to a pocketless pita. **Lavash,** a Middle Eastern bread that is traditionally rectangular, is flat and floppy. (Some lavash are round, probably in an effort to attract wrap-lovers.) For wraps, look for the thin, pliable lavash and use scissors to cut them into 8-inch squares. Thick lavash may be soaked in cold water for a few seconds to soften it, then drained and patted with kitchen towels to remove the excess water. The packages will provide specific storage instructions, but most flatbreads can be stored at room temperature for a week or so. I freeze mine. I'll buy three or four packages at a time and freeze them.

Another delicious and exotic flatbread is **injera,** which is made from teff flour and is gluten free. This Ethiopian bread has a texture similar to a buckwheat crêpe. Look for them in shops that sell African groceries or

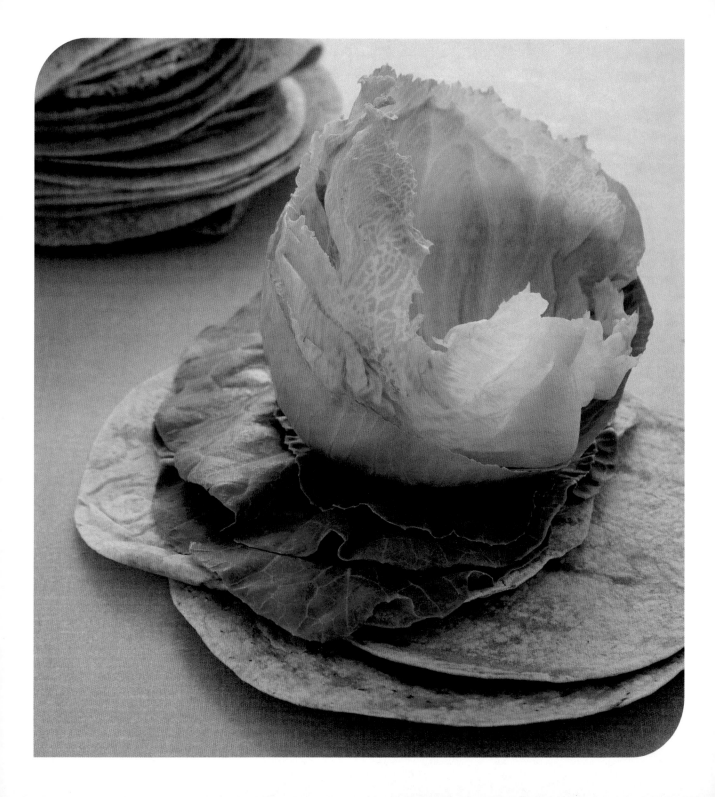

online. (I buy them from shops in Hollywood's Little Ethiopia.) Left to sit, injera quickly becomes soggy, so don't fill and wrap injera until ready to serve.

Vegetables: The healthiest choices as wrappers are leafy greens. As a general rule of thumb, the darker the greens, the higher their vitamin content. There are many good wrapper candidates in the Brassica (mustard) family, including kale, collards, and cabbage—green, red, or Chinese (napa) cabbage. These greens are fairly tough with assertive flavors, so you may wish to dip them in boiling water to make them more pliable and tame their spicy edge. The amount of time spent in the water depends on the toughness of the leaf—napa cabbage may only need a few seconds, but you may want to give kale leaves a full minute. Drain, rinse under cold water, and pat dry with kitchen towels before proceeding. If the leaf has a tough stem that gets in the way of rolling, just trim it out.

Lettuces also make great wrappers. Tender, floppy lettuces (such as butter or Bibb) fold easily and can be held in place with a wooden skewer or toothpick. Crisp lettuces (such as romaine and iceberg) often work best as cups to hold the ingredients.

Swiss chard and spinach are two more greens that can provide you with tasty and tangy wraps. Both should be submerged and washed well in cold water to remove any grit, and their thick stems removed. Your farmers' market is likely to have colorful red or rainbow chard in season, and they add lots of color to wraps. Like the brassica vegetables, chard can be boiled briefly to soften, if desired. Use the flat-leaf spinach sold in bunches and not the crinkly spinach in the bag, for the best results. If needed, overlap spinach leaves to create a larger surface for holding fillings.

Endive and its cousin radicchio have a natural cup shape that can be used to hold wrap fillings. White Belgian endive is the most common, but you may also see maroon-red endive. In addition to the common round, dark red and white radicchio, varieties with more dramatic markings are sometimes found at specialty markets.

Fennel, with its faint anise flavor, also makes an excellent serving vessel for wrap fillings. Just separate the bulb into layers to make cup shapes.

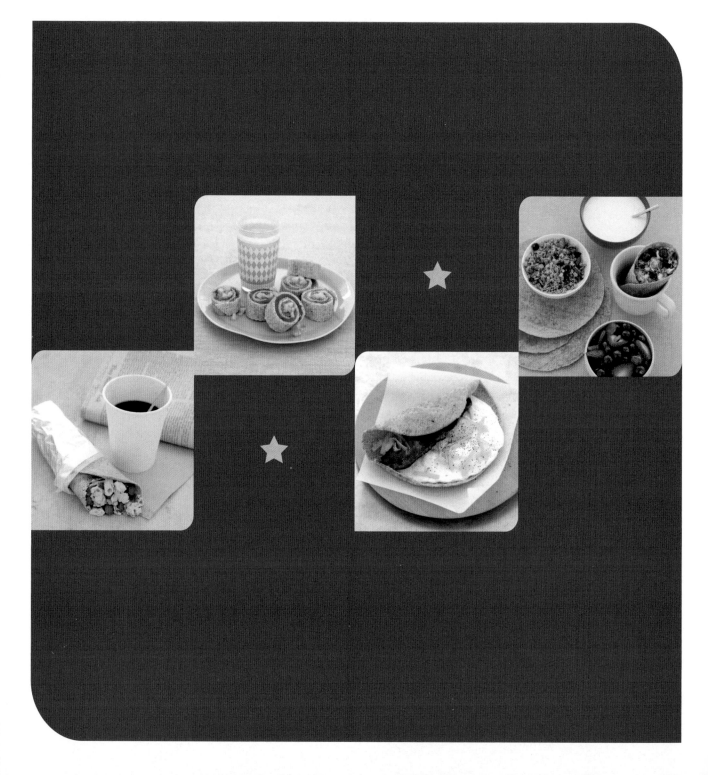

★ Breakfast Wraps

No matter how early my clients have to be on set, I insist that they eat a good breakfast before getting down to a long day's work. By a good breakfast I don't mean a huge mug of coffee with half-and-half, five spoonfuls of sugar, and a doughnut chaser from the craft table. We all need a healthy dose of real food to get our day rolling and our metabolism cranking after a good night's sleep.

When you wake up in the morning, your metabolism is slow and sluggish. You need some energy to rev it up. Aim to eat something within an hour of rising and shining. If a meal-size wrap seems too substantial first thing in the morning, eat half of it and save the other half for a midmorning snack.

Get creative when it comes to breakfast. If you feel like having a wrap made with turkey or chicken, then go for it! Lean protein is just what you need to get your metabolism up and running. Not feeling the carbs? Use vegetable leaves as wraps instead.

So roll out of bed, crank some tunes, hit the cardio machine, and chow down to get your metabolic party started Hollywood Wrap style!

Sweet Apple-Oatmeal Wraps

Oatmeal is not just deliciously warm and comforting, it is hearty, healthy, and filled with complex carbs and fiber. I love starting my day with a big bowl mixed with fruit and sometimes a scoop of protein powder. Try mixing in apple butter, a fruit spread made with no additional sugar. If you can't find apple butter at the grocery store, substitute unsweetened applesauce. And putting oatmeal in a wrap allows you to eat half at home and then the other half 3 to 4 hours later. This stick-to-your-ribs wrap is sure to get you through a hectic morning!

¼ cup apple butter

¼ cup nonfat honey–flavored yogurt

6 tablespoons honey

3 cups chopped apples

½ cup raisins

⅓ cup chopped almonds

2 teaspoons ground cinnamon

2⅔ cups vanilla soymilk or fat-free milk

2 cups instant steel-cut oats, such as McCann's

2 scoops vanilla whey protein powder

2 teaspoons vanilla extract

4 whole wheat tortillas (8-inch), plain or apple-cinnamon, warmed

1 Combine the apple butter and yogurt in a small bowl. Set aside.

2 Melt the honey in a saucepan over medium heat. Add the apples, raisins, almonds, and cinnamon. Cook until the apples are soft, 6 to 8 minutes.

3 Add the soymilk, oats, and protein powder to the saucepan and reduce the heat to low. Cook until the milk is absorbed and the oatmeal is creamy, 1 to 2 minutes. Remove from the heat and stir in the vanilla.

4 Spread each tortilla with one-quarter of the oatmeal, leaving a ½-inch border on the sides and bottom. Top each with some of the apple butter–yogurt spread. Fold the bottom end of the tortilla up and over the filling, fold in both sides, and continue rolling. Serve warm.

PER SERVING: 689 calories (98 from fat), 26 g protein, 11 g fat (1 g saturated fat), 126 g carbohydrates, 12 g fiber, 10 mg cholesterol, 428 mg sodium

How to Drop a Dress Size in Days

You are one week away from slipping into a slinky dress for a cocktail party or heading to the beach for the first time after a long winter. You need to get your skinny on ASAP. Here are 7 tried-and-true tricks Hollywood stars use the week before an important shoot or premiere to drop a dress size. Your skin will glow, your muscles will be toned, and all eyes will be on you.

1. Hydrate with H_2O. Have at least eight to ten 8-ounce glasses a day for each of the 7 days. It fills you up so you're less hungry and flushes out your system.

2. Eat asparagus frequently. It is a natural diuretic. Try Can't Beet These Wraps (page 64), Chicken-Asparagus Wraps (page 106), or Shrimp-Asparagus Rolls (page 142). Snack on blanched asparagus between meals.

3. Change your workout routine. Sweat, sweat, sweat for 45 to 60 minutes. Whatever cardio fitness you do, immediately switch it up. If you run or walk on a treadmill, hit the elliptical trainer instead. If you ride a bike, try jumping rope. Your body will sweat more when doing a new activity since it's not used to it. In fact, change up your routine every 6 weeks regardless of how fast you're trying to lose weight.

4. Eat small, but more frequent, meals. Eating snack-size portions throughout the day keeps your metabolism revved up. Have half of a Sweet Apple-Oatmeal Wrap (opposite page) for breakfast, a Greek Salad Wrap Hollywood-Style (page 67) for lunch, a protein shake (blend together protein powder, ice, water, and fruit) for an afternoon snack, and a Cobb Salad Wrap (page 102) for dinner.

5. Nix the alcohol. It's empty calories you don't need.

6. Eat lean protein. Chicken, turkey, and fish help your body eliminate excess water.

7. Avoid salt. Sodium causes your body to retain fluids, which causes bloating and swelling.

Power Fruit Wraps

Beginning the day with this cool, creamy wrap of cottage cheese, yogurt, berries, and a hit of sweet, crunchy granola gets you all the protein and vitamins you need in the morning. It's filling and can be quickly put together. Change up the strawberries and blueberries and substitute raspberries. Buy berries in season when they're inexpensive and freeze them so they're always on hand.

1 cup nonfat plain yogurt

$2/3$ cup fat-free cottage cheese

$1/4$ teaspoon vanilla extract

$3/4$ cup sliced strawberries

$3/4$ cup blueberries

$1/2$ cup seedless red grapes, sliced

$1/4$ cup diced prunes

$3/4$ cup low-fat granola

4 apple-cinnamon whole wheat tortillas
   (8-inch)

1 Combine the yogurt, cottage cheese, and vanilla in a bowl and mix together well.

2 Add the strawberries, blueberries, grapes, and prunes and mix thoroughly. Add the granola and stir well.

3 Spread one-quarter of the filling in the middle of each tortilla, leaving a $1/2$-inch border on the sides and bottom. Fold the bottom end of the tortilla up and over the filling, fold in both sides, and continue rolling.

PER SERVING: 320 calories (24 from fat), 13 g protein, 3 g fat (0 g saturated fat), 65 g carbohydrates, 6 g fiber, 5 mg cholesterol, 560 mg sodium

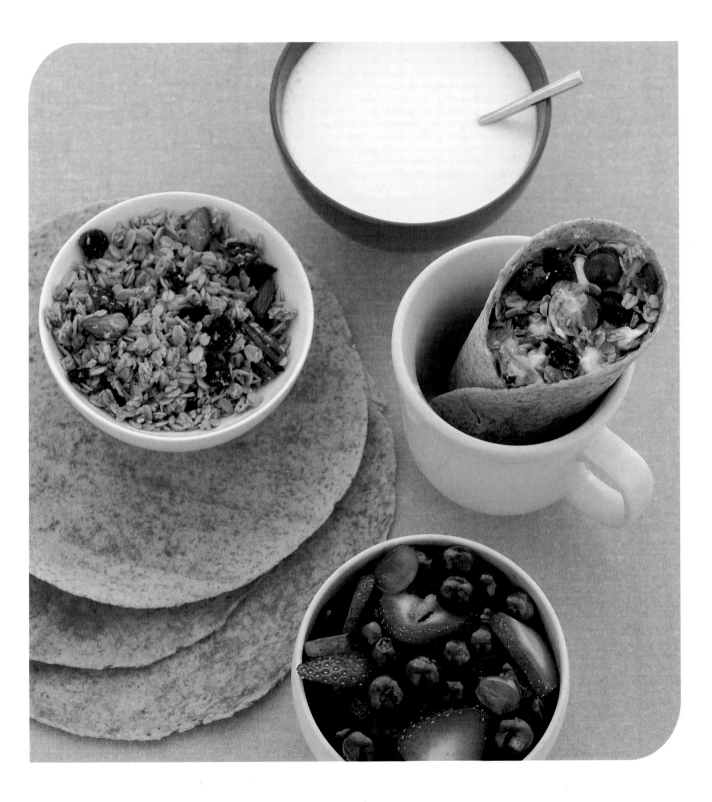

Wild Rice Wake-Up Wraps

Wild rice with your morning coffee? Absolutely! Since it's packed with protein and fiber and has a rich, nutty flavor, wild rice makes for a winning wrap when combined with fruit and topped with some yogurt. Plus, since it is botanically a grass rather than a grain, it contains twice the protein of regular rice. Wild rice takes anywhere from 40 to 50 minutes to cook, so boil it up before you hit the sack.

1 cup wild rice, rinsed

1 tablespoon maple syrup

1 teaspoon extra-virgin olive oil

1 teaspoon ground cinnamon

2 Golden Delicious apples, chopped

1 medium banana, sliced

¼ cup raisins

⅓ cup 0% honey Greek yogurt

1 teaspoon vanilla extract

2 tablespoons wheat germ

4 whole wheat tortillas (8-inch), cinnamon-flavored or plain, warmed

1 Bring the wild rice and 2 cups of water to a boil in a saucepan over high heat. Lower the heat, cover, and simmer until the rice is tender but still chewy and most of the water is absorbed, 40 to 60 minutes. Taste a few grains after 40 minutes to see if the rice is done. Drain in a colander. Cover and store in the refrigerator for up to 3 days.

2 Combine the maple syrup, oil, and cinnamon in a skillet over medium heat. Add the apples and cook until soft, 3 to 4 minutes, stirring occasionally. Stir in the cooked rice, banana, and raisins to warm them. Remove the skillet from the heat and stir in the yogurt, vanilla, and wheat germ.

3 Spread one-quarter of the rice mixture in the middle of each tortilla, leaving a ½-inch border on the sides and bottom. Fold the bottom end of the tortilla up and over the filling, fold in both sides, and continue rolling. Serve warm.

PER SERVING: 406 calories (32 from fat), 13 g protein, 4 g fat (0 g saturated fat), 85 g carbohydrates, 8 g fiber, 1 mg cholesterol, 343 mg sodium

Granola Energy Wraps

Kevin Costner loves this wrap. It makes a great lunch-box meal or an after-school snack for kids bored with ho-hum peanut butter and jelly sandwiches. Purchase all-natural nut butter with no added salt or sugar. You may even be able to have your peanut butter ground to order at your local natural food store, in which case you'll know exactly what is in it. This sweet treat is very filling, so cut it in half, eat some for breakfast, and save the rest to manage your midmorning snack attack.

3 cups sliced bananas (2 bananas)

2 cups low-fat granola

1/2 cup 0% vanilla Greek yogurt

2 teaspoons honey

1/4 cup raisins

1/4 cup chopped walnuts

1/4 cup wheat germ

1/2 cup smooth or chunky peanut butter, at room temperature

4 cinnamon-flavored whole wheat tortillas (8-inch)

1 Using a rubber spatula, mix the bananas, granola, yogurt, honey, raisins, walnuts, and wheat germ together in a bowl.

2 Spread 2 tablespoons of the peanut butter evenly on each tortilla, leaving a 1/2-inch border on the sides and bottom. Spread one-quarter of the banana mixture in the middle of each tortilla, leaving a 1/2-inch border on the sides and bottom. Fold the bottom end of the tortilla up and over the filling, fold in both sides, and continue rolling. Serve.

PER SERVING: 686 calories (229 from fat), 22 g protein, 25 g fat (4 g saturated fat), 103 g carbohydrates, 11 g fiber, 0 mg cholesterol, 615 mg sodium

Set Up for Success

Work out before you leave the house or, if you have a gym membership, get there first thing in the morning. In all my years as a trainer, I've learned that if you don't get it out of the way before you start the day, it's not happenin'. Something is always better than nothing. Even if you only work up a sweat 15 minutes a day, it all adds up, and by the end of the week, you'll see the physical results.

Frittata *of* Champions Wraps

A frittata is just like a quiche, but without the fattening crust! Slice it into wedges and roll it in a tortilla for an on-the-go breakfast, lunch, or dinner. A crispy spinach salad makes a fabulous accompaniment to this eggy delight.

1 teaspoon extra-virgin olive oil

1 cup thinly sliced red onion

¼ cup chopped red bell pepper

1 teaspoon chopped rosemary

1 cup chopped spinach

2 teaspoons minced garlic

1 can (15 ounces) cannellini beans, rinsed and drained

2 eggs

5 egg whites

1 teaspoon freshly ground black pepper

4 ounces fat-free feta cheese, crumbled

4 garden veggie or whole wheat tortillas (8-inch), warmed

1 Preheat the broiler.

2 Heat the oil in a broilerproof medium skillet over medium heat. Add the onion, bell pepper, and rosemary and cook for 5 to 6 minutes, stirring occasionally. Cover and cook until the onion and pepper are translucent, another 5 to 6 minutes. Add the spinach and garlic and cook just until the spinach is wilted, about 1 minute. Remove the skillet from the heat. Stir in the beans.

3 Whisk the whole eggs, egg whites, and black pepper together in a bowl. Stir in half of the feta. Add the sautéed vegetables and beans to the eggs and stir well to combine.

4 Coat the same skillet used to cook the spinach with cooking spray. Add the egg-vegetable mixture to the skillet and cook over medium heat until the vegetables are gently browned and soft, 3 to 4 minutes. Remove from the heat and sprinkle the remaining feta on top.

5 Wrap the skillet handle with foil if it's not broilerproof. Place the skillet under the broiler a medium distance from the heat for 7 to 8 minutes, until the frittata is lightly browned on top and firm.

6 Remove the pan from the oven and turn the frittata out onto a cutting board. Cut into 4 wedges. Put one wedge in the middle of each tortilla. Fold the bottom end of the tortilla up and over the filling, fold in both sides, and continue rolling. Serve hot.

PER SERVING: 320 calories (52 from fat), 23 g protein, 6 g fat (1 g saturated fat), 43 g carbohydrates, 7 g fiber, 110 mg cholesterol, 874 mg sodium

Eat Your Fruits and Vegetables

Doctor's orders are five servings of fruits and vegetables per day, and it's really worth it to your health and your body to listen! Fruits and vegetables are low-cal and loaded with fiber, minerals, and vitamins. Here are some tips that will help you increase your intake:

★ Add sprouts, lettuce, tomatoes, and cucumbers to wraps and sandwiches.

★ Add berries, sliced apples, and pears to green salads.

★ Add peppers, carrots, peas, corn, and beans to salads.

★ Make a soy protein shake with fruit to start your day. Use fat-free milk, a scoop of protein powder, a handful of berries, and ice.

★ Use cooked and pureed fruits—apples, pears, and berries—as sauces to top shrimp, chicken, and other protein dishes.

★ Add chopped kale or spinach to pasta sauces.

Southwestern Scramble Wraps

★ :: **MAKES 4**

I love Southwestern food, but super-fatty cheeses and sour cream don't love me, and they won't love you, either. A lot of Southwestern favorites, like breakfast burritos, are loaded with grease and unhealthy calories, sometimes as much as 1,200 per meal. If your entire daily-allotted calorie count is 2,000 . . . well, you do the math. Try this low-fat, low-cal egg and cheese scramble wrap instead. It's a big hit with my Hollywood clients.

8 egg whites

2 eggs

3 tablespoons chopped cilantro

$3/4$ cup canned pinto beans, rinsed and drained

$1/3$ cup chopped scallions

$1/3$ cup shredded fat-free Cheddar cheese

$1/3$ cup Salsa Picante (page 39)

$1/4$ cup fat-free sour cream

4 cilantro-flavored whole wheat tortillas (8-inch), warmed

1 Whisk together the egg whites, whole eggs, and cilantro in a bowl. Put the beans, scallions, cheese, salsa, and sour cream in another bowl and stir well to combine.

2 Heat a skillet over medium heat and coat lightly with cooking spray. Add the egg mixture and cook for 2 to 3 minutes. Stir in the bean mixture and continue to cook until the eggs are scrambled to desired doneness.

3 Spread one-quarter of the filling in the middle of each tortilla, leaving a $1/2$-inch border on the sides and bottom. Fold the bottom end of the tortilla up and over the filling, fold in both sides, and continue rolling. Serve.

PER SERVING: 277 calories (42 from fat), 21 g protein, 5 g fat (1 g saturated fat), 38 g carbohydrates, 6 g fiber, 109 mg cholesterol, 637 mg sodium

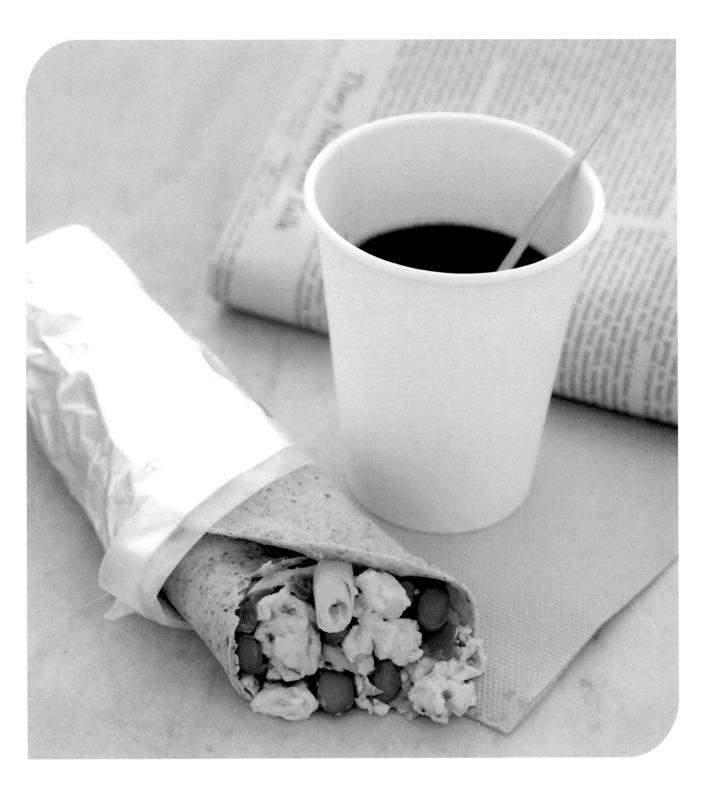

Huevos Rancheros Wraps

Huevos Rancheros is a hearty, flavorful breakfast dish popular in the Southwest, but the traditional ingredients will pack on the pounds. This healthy take brings all the sizzle while still keeping you Hollywood skinny! These wraps aren't portable, but they're great for brunch or even dinner at home. Make sure you choose refried beans that contain no lard and are fat free, and feel free to add fat-free Cheddar or chopped sweet onions for an extra burst. *Olé!*

1 cup fat-free (or vegetarian) refried beans, warmed

4 Nopaltilla tortillas (5$\frac{1}{2}$-inch), warmed

4 eggs

$\frac{1}{2}$ cup crumbled fat-free feta cheese

$\frac{1}{2}$ cup salsa verde

$\frac{1}{4}$ cup fat-free sour cream

$\frac{1}{2}$ Hass avocado, thinly sliced

1 Spread the refried beans on the tortillas. Set aside.

2 Heat a skillet over medium-high heat. Coat with cooking spray. Slide 2 eggs into the pan, turn the heat down to low, and cook the eggs until the whites are opaque and the yolks are cooked to desired doneness. Using a spatula, remove the eggs and place one on top of each tortilla. Cook the remaining 2 eggs the same way.

3 Top each tortilla and egg with feta, salsa verde, sour cream, and avocado. Fold and serve warm.

PER SERVING: 247 calories (75 from fat), 16 g protein, 8 g fat (2 g saturated fat), 27 g carbohydrates, 6 g fiber, 216 mg cholesterol, 639 mg sodium

Kick Start Egg
and Sausage
Wraps

Chicken-apple sausage is a delicious, lower-fat treat that's even better paired with eggs. And talk about protein! This will definitely kick-start your day, complement your workout, and help build muscle. To avoid wasting a ton of yolks, purchase pure egg whites in cartons from the dairy case. They're super low-cal and totally fat free. One-quarter cup liquid egg whites equals the whites of two large eggs.

2 low-fat chicken-apple sausages, cut into $\frac{1}{4}$**-inch pieces**

4 eggs

16 egg whites

$\frac{1}{4}$ **cup crumbled fat-free feta cheese**

4 whole wheat tortillas (8-inch), apple-cinnamon or plain

10 large basil leaves, chopped

1 Coat a skillet with cooking spray and heat over medium-high heat. Add the sausages and cook, stirring occasionally, until browned. Drain the sausages on paper towels.

2 Whisk together the whole eggs and egg whites in a bowl. Coat the skillet with more cooking spray if necessary, add the eggs, and scramble. Just before the eggs are cooked to desired doneness, turn off the heat and stir in the feta.

3 Spread one-quarter of the filling in the middle of each tortilla, leaving a $\frac{1}{2}$-inch border on the sides and bottom. Sprinkle with the basil. Fold the bottom end of the tortilla up and over the filling, fold in both sides, and continue rolling. Serve.

PER SERVING: 329 calories (79 from fat), 32 g protein, 9 g fat (2 g saturated fat), 31 g carbohydrates, 3 g fiber, 233 mg cholesterol, 858 mg sodium

Bacon, Egg, *and* Cheese Wraps

Usually served on a big, fluffy, carborific roll, this breakfast sandwich is the to-go choice at delis and coffee shops everywhere. My Hollywood version is made with turkey bacon, a combination of whole eggs and egg whites, and fat-free cheese on a wrap for a much lighter, much healthier on-the-go breakfast choice.

4 turkey bacon strips

4 eggs

4 egg whites

2 whole wheat pitas (8-inch), split horizontally and warmed

½ cup shredded fat-free Cheddar cheese

1 Cook the turkey bacon in a nonstick skillet over medium heat until crisp. Drain the bacon on paper towels. Discard all but 1 teaspoon of the fat from the skillet.

2 Cook the eggs for each wrap separately: Break 1 whole egg into a dish and add 1 egg white (save the yolk for another use). Slide the egg mixture into the heated skillet. Cook until the whites turn opaque. For a well-cooked yolk, cover the pan with a lid for 30 seconds. (Using this method rather than flipping them means there's less risk of breaking the yolk.)

3 When the egg is done to your satisfaction, use a spatula to transfer it to a warmed pita. Top with 1 strip of turkey bacon and 2 tablespoons of the cheese. Fold the bottom end of the pita up and over the filling, fold in both sides, and continue rolling.

4 Repeat the steps with the remaining whole eggs and whites, turkey bacon, and cheese, adding ½ teaspoon of fat to the pan as needed to cook each egg. Serve immediately.

PER SERVING: 286 calories (124 from fat), 22 g protein, 14 g fat (3 g saturated fat), 20 g carbohydrates, 2 g fiber, 240 mg cholesterol, 739 mg sodium

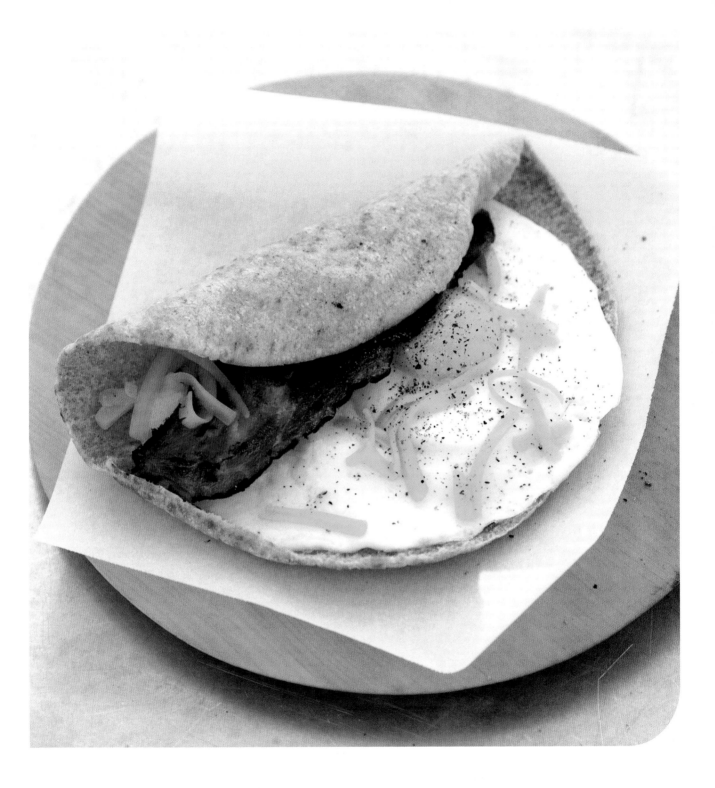

Scrambled Tofu *and* Eggs *with* Salsa

★ :: **MAKES 4**

This scrambled tofu-and-egg wrap provides plenty of protein, and the fragrant turmeric and spicy salsa will wake your sleepy body and mind right up. Turmeric, a spice used in Indian cooking, has been shown to have antioxidant, anti-inflammatory, antibacterial, and fat-burning properties. Consider using more of it in your cooking.

4 egg whites

2 eggs

⅛ teaspoon turmeric

6 ounces extra-firm tofu, drained and cubed

¼ cup fat-free shredded Cheddar cheese

½ cup Salsa Picante (recipe follows)

4 whole wheat tortillas (8-inch), warmed

1 Whisk together the egg whites, whole eggs, and turmeric in a bowl. Set aside.

2 Coat a nonstick skillet with cooking spray and heat the skillet over medium-high heat.

3 Add the tofu and cook, stirring occasionally, until the tofu is browned, about 5 minutes. Keep the tofu in cubes or break them up, as you wish.

4 Lower the heat to medium. Add the egg mixture to the tofu and continue to cook, stirring constantly with a wooden spoon. When the eggs begin to scramble, stir in the cheese and salsa and continue cooking until the eggs are done.

5 Spread one-quarter of the filling in the middle of each tortilla, leaving a ½-inch border on the sides and bottom. Fold the bottom end of the tortilla up and over the filling, fold in both sides, and continue rolling. Serve warm.

PER SERVING: 244 calories (62 from fat), 18 g protein, 7 g fat (1 g saturated fat), 29 g carbohydrates, 4 g fiber, 107 mg cholesterol, 501 mg sodium

SALSA PICANTE

MAKES ABOUT 2 CUPS

Homemade salsa is simple to whip up, and you can control the heat to taste. Although salsa is usually served as a condiment, it is filled with so much flavor and healthy veggies that it could be a wrap filling on its own! If you don't want to make your own salsa, choose carefully at the grocery store. Spring for salsas low in sugar and sodium.

4 tomatoes, chopped

1 jalapeño pepper, seeded and minced

⅓ cup diced red onion

¼ cup chopped cilantro

2 garlic cloves, finely minced

2 scallions, finely chopped

Pinch of cayenne pepper

Juice of 1 lime

Coarse sea salt and freshly ground black pepper, to taste

Combine all the ingredients in a large bowl. Mix thoroughly and set aside for 45 minutes to 1 hour so the flavors can meld.

PER SERVING (2 tablespoons): 9 calories (1 from fat), 0 g protein, 0 g fat (0 g saturated fat), 2 g carbohydrates, 0.5 g fiber, 0 mg cholesterol, 27 mg sodium

Exercise Is the Best Shrink in the World

Working out is good for your self-esteem. You just feel better. You walk taller. No, really, it's true! I was painfully skinny as a kid and constantly teased. As my body began to mature, nothing made me feel more powerful than lifting weights and watching my body change. I was no longer that skinny kid; I became that attractive woman!

Exercise is an antidepressant. Because exercise releases your body's endorphins (neurotransmitters that resemble opiates and that give you that exercise "high"), it makes you feel better mentally and emotionally.

Smoking Salmon Wraps

Smoked salmon is deliciously rich and has amazing health benefits. It's a great source of lean protein and contains omega-3 fats, which can lower the risk of heart disease and decrease blood lipids. This wrap is a no-cook no-brainer; just roll and go! And it makes a great brunch dish or party appetizer. Just remember, because smoked salmon is salty, you should watch your salt intake at other meals during the day and wash your wrap down with plenty of H_2O.

½ cup fat-free cream cheese

2 tablespoons chopped capers

1 teaspoon dried dillweed

4 whole wheat tortillas (8-inch)

8 ounces smoked salmon

⅔ cup peeled, diced cucumber

2 tablespoons diced red onion

1 Combine the cream cheese, capers, and dill in a small bowl and stir until blended.

2 Spread each tortilla with one-quarter of the cream cheese mixture, leaving a ½-inch border on the sides and bottom. Top each with the salmon, cucumber, and onion. Fold the bottom end of the tortilla up and over the filling, fold in both sides, and continue rolling. Serve.

PER SERVING: 359 calories (76 from fat), 43 g protein, 8 g fat (2 g saturated fat), 29 g carbohydrates, 3 g fiber, 90 mg cholesterol, 676 mg sodium

Your Mother Was Right!

No ifs, ands, or buts about it: Breakfast is the most important meal of the day. When you wake up, your body and your metabolism have been in rest mode for the past 7 or more hours. (Women's metabolisms slow down after only 3 hours without food, and men's slow down after 5 hours.) Eating speeds your metabolism back up, and doing so right when you rise and shine literally breaks the fast your body has been on overnight. If you wait until later in the day to eat a healthy meal, you slow down your own metabolism.

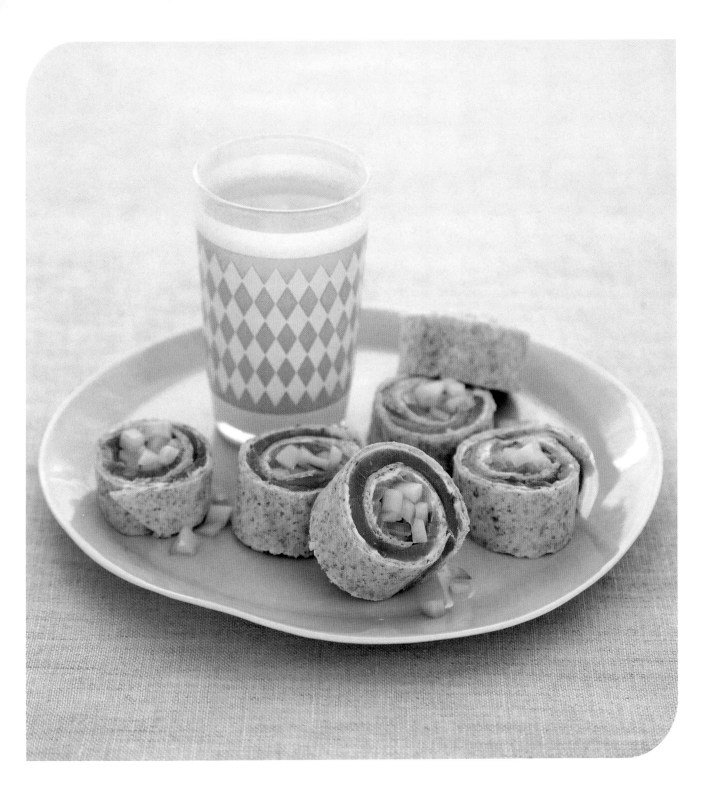

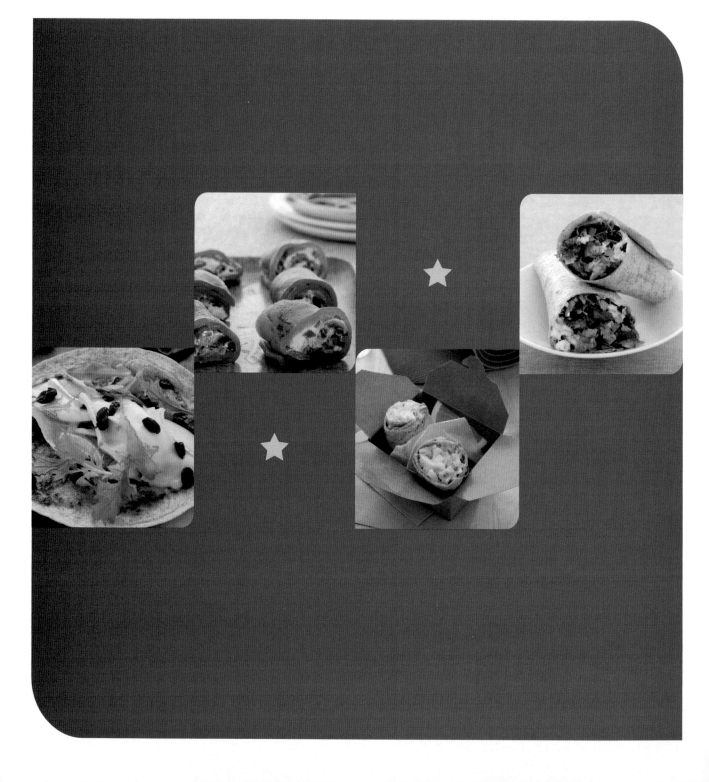

★ Vegetarian Wraps

Many of my Hollywood clients are vegetarians—some because they are ardent animal lovers, others because they want to eliminate saturated fat from their diets. Saturated fats occur naturally in meat and dairy products like beef, pork, lamb, poultry, eggs, butter, and cheese, and also in palm, coconut, and other tropical oils. These fats increase the risk of heart disease by elevating your total and LDL ("bad") cholesterol in your blood. Other harmful fats with a similar health downside include trans fats: hydrogenated vegetable oils found in shortening, margarine, and processed foods such as baked goods, cookies, crackers, and snack foods.

To avoid heart problems and diseases like diabetes, it's simple: Eat less saturated fat. No need to go completely veg. Just start by eating meat-free meals one or two days a week. Know that on Mondays and Thursdays, for example, you'll be eating soy-based proteins (like tofu and tempeh), grains, veggies, fruits, and nuts with the occasional low-fat dairy products and eggs. If you find that you prefer and feel better eating this way, then go for it on other days of the week.

In this chapter, you'll find lots of ideas for healthy, satisfying vegetarian wraps. Use them as a jumping-off point for getting crafty with your own skinny creations.

Red Pepper, Mushroom, *and* Goat Cheese Wraps

Want to wrap your lunch in something new? This recipe uses roasted peppers (available in jars). Fresh or soft goat cheese is super flavorful, and is lower in fat and calories than some cheeses made with cow's milk, especially if you choose a low-fat variety (Coach Farm makes a lovely one). Even if you can't find low-fat goat cheese, this wrap is still wicked healthy—and the combination of flavors will knock your socks off.

1 tablespoon extra-virgin olive oil

½ large onion, sliced

8 ounces mushrooms, sliced

⅓ cup balsamic vinegar

8 roasted red peppers (patted dry if packed in oil)

8 ounces fresh goat cheese, at room temperature

1 Heat the oil in a skillet over medium heat. Add the onion and cook for 3 to 5 minutes. Add the mushrooms and cook until the onions are soft, browned, and slightly translucent, another 10 to 12 minutes. Add the vinegar to the skillet and stir to loosen any browned bits on the bottom of the skillet and to coat the vegetables.

2 Arrange 2 roasted peppers, slightly overlapping one another, on a work surface to make a "wrap." Spread one-quarter of the goat cheese on each roasted pepper "wrap." Top with the mushroom mixture, roll up, and serve.

PER SERVING: 242 calories (141 from fat), 13 g protein, 16 g fat (9 g saturated fat), 14 g carbohydrates, 3 g fiber, 26 mg cholesterol, 277 mg sodium

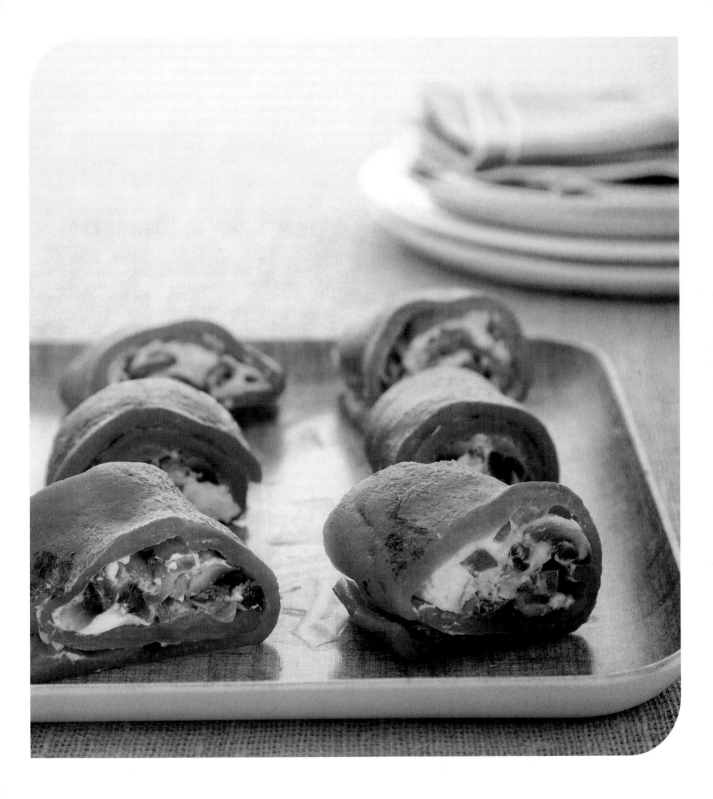

Mediterranean Salad Wraps

As long as you've got beans, you will never be without a healthy source of protein. Chickpeas are firm with a slight nutty flavor and add texture to any salad, chili, or wrap. Instead of reaching for a bag of greasy potato chips, crisp some chickpeas in a pan with some spices for snacking. You can also use the herb dressing in this recipe on your favorite salads or as a dip with sliced veggies.

3 tablespoons extra-virgin olive oil

1½ tablespoons fresh lemon juice

2 garlic cloves, chopped

¾ teaspoon dried oregano

¼ teaspoon freshly ground black pepper

1 can (15 ounces) chickpeas, rinsed and drained

1 cucumber, peeled, halved lengthwise, and sliced crosswise

6 cherry tomatoes

¼ red onion, chopped

¼ cup crumbled fat-free feta cheese

4 butter lettuce leaves

1 Whisk together the oil, lemon juice, garlic, oregano, and black pepper in a large bowl.

2 Add the chickpeas, cucumber, tomatoes, red onion, and feta to the bowl. Toss well and refrigerate for 30 minutes to blend the flavors.

3 Spoon the salad onto the lettuce leaves, roll up, and serve.

PER SERVING: 195 calories (108 from fat), 7 g protein, 12 g fat (1.5 g saturated fat), 16 g carbohydrates, 4 g fiber, 1 mg cholesterol, 177 mg sodium

Caponata *and* Feta Wraps

Caponata, a Sicilian ratatouille, is filled with healthy veggies, but it's often swimming in olive oil. In this leaner version, the vegetables retain their shape and flavor, and a sprinkle of feta adds some protein. Caponata can be made ahead and refrigerated for several days. You can also spoon the caponata into crunchy fresh fennel or endive leaves.

2 teaspoons extra-virgin olive oil

4 cups peeled, cubed eggplant

2 cups chopped onions

1 cup chopped green bell pepper

1 cup chopped red bell pepper

1 cup chopped celery

2 garlic cloves, minced

¼ cup chopped fresh basil

2 tablespoons chopped parsley

½ teaspoon chopped fresh oregano or pinch of dried

4 tomatoes, chopped

½ cup crumbled fat-free feta cheese

4 large romaine lettuce leaves, center ribs cut out

1 Heat the oil in a skillet over medium heat. Add the eggplant, onions, peppers, celery, garlic, basil, parsley, and oregano. Cook, stirring occasionally, until the vegetables are soft, about 15 minutes.

2 Remove the skillet from the heat and stir in the tomatoes and cheese. Let cool for 15 minutes or to room temperature.

3 Spoon one-quarter of the caponata into the center of each lettuce leaf. Carefully roll up and serve.

PER SERVING: 148 calories (28 from fat), 9 g protein, 3 g fat (0.5 g saturated fat), 24 g carbohydrates, 8 g fiber, 3 mg cholesterol, 210 mg sodium

Caprese Melts

These pizza-like wraps are a twist on the traditional Caprese salad: slices of juicy tomato and cool mozzarella sprinkled with fresh basil. I like to add fresh garlic to give them even more of a kick. Heat the wraps in the oven just until the cheese is melted to gooey perfection. For a true Italian-style family meal, kick off these wraps with an antipasto platter of salad or a mixture of roasted red peppers, sun-dried tomatoes (not packed in oil), fresh figs, and olives.

4 garlic-flavored whole wheat tortillas (8-inch)

6 tablespoons shredded part-skim mozzarella cheese

¼ cup sliced roasted red peppers

4 plum tomatoes, sliced

12 basil leaves

1 teaspoon minced garlic

1 Preheat the oven to 350°F.

2 Arrange the tortillas on a baking sheet. Top each one with one-quarter of the cheese, peppers, tomatoes, basil leaves, and garlic, leaving a ½-inch border on the sides and bottom.

3 Fold the bottom end of the tortilla up and over the filling, fold in both sides, and continue rolling. Bake for 4 to 6 minutes, until the cheese is melted. Serve hot.

PER SERVING: 179 calories (33 from fat), 7 g protein, 4 g fat (1 g saturated fat), 29 g carbohydrates, 4 g fiber, 0 mg cholesterol, 417 mg sodium

AB&Js

Peanut butter's delish, but why not snazz up the traditional PB&J with another rich, creamy member of the nut butter family? These wraps combine organic almond butter, cream cheese, and fruit spread.

2 tablespoons almond butter

4 whole wheat tortillas (8-inch), warmed

4 tablespoons fat-free cream cheese, at room temperature

2 tablespoons all-fruit spread

2 bananas, sliced

1 Spread one-quarter of the almond butter in the middle of each tortilla, leaving a $\frac{1}{2}$-inch border on the sides and bottom.

2 Top with the cream cheese, fruit spread, and bananas. Fold the bottom end of the tortilla up and over the filling, fold in both sides, and continue rolling. Serve.

PER SERVING: 267 calories (59 from fat), 8 g protein, 7 g fat (1 g saturated fat), 47 g carbohydrates, 5 g fiber, 1 mg cholesterol, 447 mg sodium

Gut Busters

★ Take the stairs instead of the elevator whenever possible.

★ If you sit at a desk all day, do this tush squeeze a few times. Sit up straight in your chair, pull your abs in tight, and squeeze your booty for 2 to 3 minutes! Relax. Repeat 20 times. Do this at least three times during your workday and you'll be as bootylicious as Ms. Beyoncé! Just make sure no one's looking—don't want the boss to see you wiggling in your chair!

★ Do you drive to work? Park three to four blocks from the office and walk briskly the rest of the way. This will elevate your heart rate and increase energy levels. You may be surprised how these daily jaunts to and from the workplace add to your daily exercise count of 30 minutes per day.

★ Going out to lunch? Take the long way—no shortcuts—and walk those few extra blocks before and after you eat.

★ Keep walking shoes at the office, put them on at lunch, and head out the door for a 30-minute walk 5 days a week. Chow down when you get back. A friend of mine lost 15 pounds over the course of a year just by being persistent with her walking regimen. Walking is easy on your joints, great for your heart, and key to a fabulous bod!

Curried Egg Salad Wraps

Always have some hard-boiled eggs in the fridge so you can put together this light, yummy wrap right after a workout. Discarding half of the yolks gets rid of some unnecessary fat, and you are left with the protein-packed whites to pair with creamy, fat-free mayo and the zesty combo of spices that gets this satisfying salad snack rave reviews.

¼ cup fat-free mayonnaise

1 teaspoon fresh lime juice

1 teaspoon curry powder

1 teaspoon Dijon mustard

Freshly ground white pepper

8 hard-boiled eggs, peeled

¼ cup diced celery

¼ cup diced red onion

¼ cup chopped cilantro

4 pieces (8 x 8-inch) whole wheat lavash

1 Whisk together the mayonnaise, lime juice, curry powder, mustard, and white pepper to taste in a medium bowl.

2 Halve the eggs and discard 4 of the yolks. Add the remaining yolks and whites to the bowl with the mayonnaise mixture and mash with a fork. Add the celery, red onion, and cilantro and mix well.

3 Spread one-quarter of the egg salad in the middle of each lavash, leaving a ¹/₂-inch border on the sides and bottom. Fold the bottom end of the lavash up and over the filling, fold in both sides, and continue rolling. Serve.

PER SERVING: 198 calories (66 from fat), 13 g protein, 7 g fat (2 g saturated fat), 22 g carbohydrates, 4 g fiber, 214 mg cholesterol, 296 mg sodium

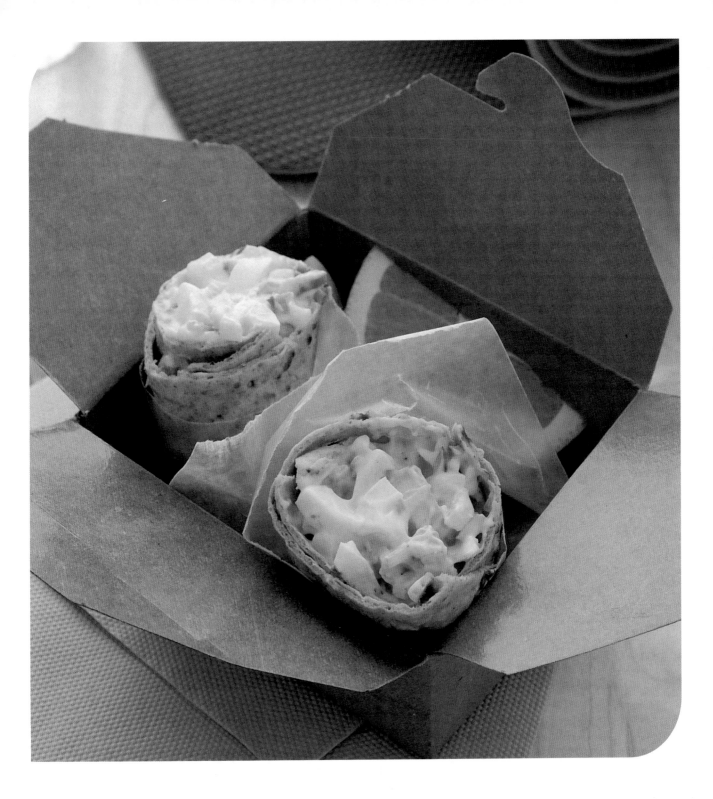

Spinach Pizza
Pie Rolls

I bet some of you (like me) could eat cheesy pizza every day. Yet we all know that one greasy take-out slice can undo an entire day's workout. Try my quick, healthy pizza fix instead; you'll be amazed at just how good it is. Serve it to adults and/or hungry kids with a big green salad and fresh melon slices for dessert.

2 whole wheat pitas, split horizontally

½ cup Marinara Sauce (recipe follows)

2 cups chopped spinach

2 cups sliced mushrooms

2 cups shredded fat-free mozzarella cheese

1   Preheat the oven to 350°F.

2   Arrange the pita halves on a baking sheet. Spoon 2 tablespoons of sauce onto each pita half, then top with the spinach, mushrooms, and cheese.

3   Bake for 5 to 7 minutes, or until the cheese has melted. Roll up and serve hot.

PER SERVING: 161 calories (1 from fat), 24 g protein, 1 g fat (0 g saturated fat), 19 g carbohydrates, 7 g fiber, 10 mg cholesterol, 629 mg sodium

MARINARA SAUCE

MAKES 6 CUPS

This hearty, antioxidant-rich red sauce contains no oil! Canned tomato products often contain a good dose of salt, so if sodium consumption is a dietary issue for you, crush, puree, and stew fresh tomatoes for this recipe.

1 can (28 ounces) whole peeled tomatoes

1 can (28 ounces) crushed tomatoes

1 can (28 ounces) tomato puree, preferably a no-salt-added brand

2 garlic cloves, minced

¼ cup chopped parsley

¼ cup chopped basil

Salt and freshly ground black pepper, to taste

1 Combine all the ingredients in a large pot and bring to a simmer over medium heat. Reduce the heat to low and cook for 1 hour, stirring occasionally.

2 For a smoother texture, cool the sauce and blend to desired consistency. Store in the refrigerator for 3 days or freeze for 2 months.

PER SERVING (1 cup): 126 calories (6 from fat), 6 g protein, 1 g fat (0 g saturated fat), 27 g carbohydrates, 6 g fiber, 0 mg cholesterol, 522 mg sodium

Tips for Cutting Out, Down, and Back When Cooking

★ If a recipe calls for cream, substitute fat-free milk or soymilk.

★ Use nonfat yogurt, instead of heavy cream, to add creaminess to soups.

★ Use fat-free sour cream, nonfat plain Greek yogurt, and reduced-fat cheeses instead of their full-fat counterparts.

★ Switch to fat-free mayonnaise instead of the regular kind. Vegans can use Spectrum Light Canola Mayo (eggless) or Vegenaise.

★ Substitute low-fat, low-sodium chicken stock, no-sugar-added fruit juice, or wine for oil when sautéing.

★ Substitute extra-lean ground turkey breast in recipes that call for ground beef.

Buffalo Tempeh Wraps *with* Blue Cheese Dressing

Inspired by Buffalo chicken wings, these wraps are made with nutty and nutritious tempeh and still pack an oozy, hot-sauce kick. Hailing from Indonesia, tempeh is made with beans, usually soy, that have been fermented and pressed into cakes. A hint of pungent blue cheese is all that's needed in these wraps; don't overdo it and wreck your plan to be Hollywood skinny!

2 tablespoons crumbled blue cheese

¼ cup 0% plain Greek yogurt

1 teaspoon extra-virgin olive oil

8 ounces tempeh, cut into 4 equal squares

1½ teaspoons hot sauce

1 tablespoon maple syrup

1 tablespoon fresh lemon juice

4 jalapeño/cilantro-flavored whole wheat tortillas (8-inch)

2 cups mixed greens

1 Whisk together the blue cheese and yogurt in a bowl. Set aside.

2 Heat the oil in a skillet over medium-high heat. Add the tempeh and cook, turning occasionally, until browned. Reduce the heat and stir in the hot sauce, maple syrup, and lemon juice. Continue to cook until most of the sauce is absorbed by the tempeh. Watch the tempeh carefully so it doesn't burn. Once it starts to become darker in color, it's done.

3 Top each tortilla with one-quarter of the tempeh. Top with the greens and dressing. Fold the bottom end of each tortilla up and over the filling, fold in both sides, and continue rolling. Serve.

PER SERVING: 294 calories (76 from fat), 19 g protein, 8 g fat (2 g saturated fat), 39 g carbohydrates, 8 g fiber, 3 mg cholesterol, 448 mg sodium

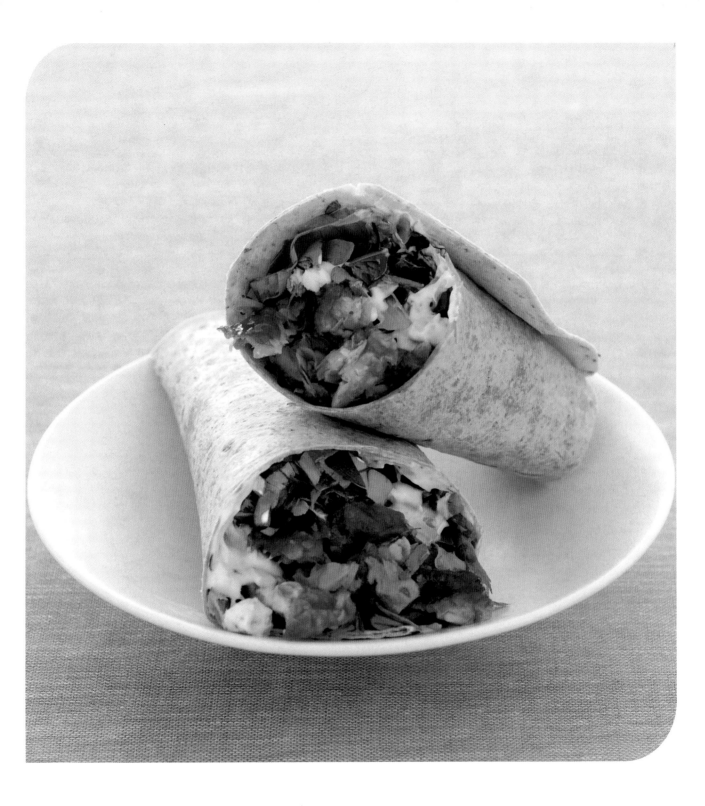

Tex-Mex Burritos

Who needs meat when you can wrap up a zesty, totally filling veggie burrito? This one is loaded with peppers, zucchini, beans, and avocado for a kick that will keep you going afternoon or evening. Be sure to buy fat-free refried beans. Some brands are made with lard, an unhealthy saturated fat.

1/4 cup Salsa Picante (page 39)

1/4 cup fat-free sour cream

2 teaspoons extra-virgin olive oil

2 red, green, or yellow bell peppers, cut into 1/2-inch-wide strips

2 medium zucchini, cut into thin strips

1 can (15 1/2 ounces) fat-free refried beans

4 whole wheat tortillas (8-inch), plain or spinach-flavored, warmed

1 Hass avocado, sliced

1 Stir together the salsa and sour cream in a small bowl. Set aside.

2 Heat the oil in a nonstick skillet over medium heat. Add the peppers and zucchini, and cook until the vegetables are soft and slightly browned, 5 to 7 minutes.

3 Spread one-quarter of the refried beans in the middle of each tortilla, leaving a 1/2-inch border on the sides and bottom. Top each tortilla with one-quarter of the sautéed vegetables, avocado slices, and 2 table-spoons of the salsa mixture. Fold the bottom end of the tortilla up and over the filling, fold in both sides, and continue rolling. Serve.

PER SERVING: 363 calories (85 from fat), 14 g protein, 9 g fat (1 g saturated fat), 56 g carbohydrates, 11 g fiber, 3 mg cholesterol, 759 mg sodium

Butternut Squash Enchiladas

These baked, squash-filled wraps are absolutely bursting with flavor: creamy cheese, fragrant cinnamon and nutmeg, and savory tomato sauce. You can buy butternut squash already peeled and cubed in many produce departments. Since you don't have to prep the squash yourself, use those 5 minutes to do some leg-toning lunges instead!

2 cups small chunks butternut squash

$\frac{1}{2}$ onion, chopped

4 ounces fat-free cream cheese

1 tablespoon molasses

2 teaspoons ground cinnamon

1 teaspoon grated nutmeg

4 whole wheat tortillas (8-inch)

$\frac{1}{2}$ cup Marinara Sauce (page 53)

$\frac{1}{2}$ cup shredded part-skim mozzarella cheese

2 tablespoons chopped parsley

1 Bring a saucepan of water to a boil. Add the squash and cook until tender when pierced with a fork, 20 to 25 minutes. Drain.

2 Meanwhile, heat a small skillet over medium-low heat. Coat with cooking spray and add the onion. Cook until the onions are soft and brown, 12 to 15 minutes. Preheat the oven to 350°F.

3 Add the onion, cream cheese, molasses, cinnamon, and nutmeg to the squash. Using a potato masher, mash the mixture until smooth.

4 Arrange the tortillas on a baking sheet. Spread one-quarter of the squash mixture over each tortilla, leaving a $\frac{1}{2}$-inch border all around. Top each with 2 tablespoons each marinara and mozzarella.

5 Bake for 10 minutes, or until the cheese melts. Remove and sprinkle with the parsley. Fold the bottom end of the tortilla up and over the filling, fold in both sides, and continue rolling. Serve hot.

PER SERVING: 267 calories (41 from fat), 13 g protein, 5 g fat (2 g saturated fat), 46 g carbohydrates, 6 g fiber, 11 mg cholesterol, 644 mg sodium

Summer Squash Wraps

Yellow summer squash and zucchini abound in gardens and at farmers' markets during the warm months of the year. Good thing they are delicious and super easy to cook with! Bake them in strips so they are soft and pliable, and use them for these wraps or in salads with a sprinkling of feta or Parmesan cheese.

1 medium zucchini, cut lengthwise into $\frac{1}{4}$-inch-thick slices and then quartered

1 yellow summer squash, cut lengthwise into $\frac{1}{4}$-inch-thick slices and then quartered

$\frac{1}{4}$ cup crumbled fat-free feta cheese

$\frac{1}{4}$ cup sun-dried (not oil-packed) tomatoes, diced

$\frac{1}{4}$ cup chopped walnuts

1 Preheat the oven to 350°F. Coat a baking sheet with cooking spray. Arrange the squash cut side up on the baking sheet and bake for 15 minutes, until softened and cooked through.

2 Mix the feta, tomatoes, and walnuts together in a small bowl. Sprinkle the feta mixture on top of the squash strips. Roll up and serve.

PER SERVING: 84 calories (45 from fat), 5 g protein, 5 g fat (0.5 g saturated fat), 7 g carbohydrates, 2 g fiber, 1 mg cholesterol, 162 mg sodium

Pump Up the Jam

Listening to your favorite tunes while you run, bike, or lift can keep you going harder and longer. Download high-energy music onto your iPod or, if you're working out with a friend, play music from the '60s and '70s and try to guess the band. It will make a 30-minute workout whiz by.

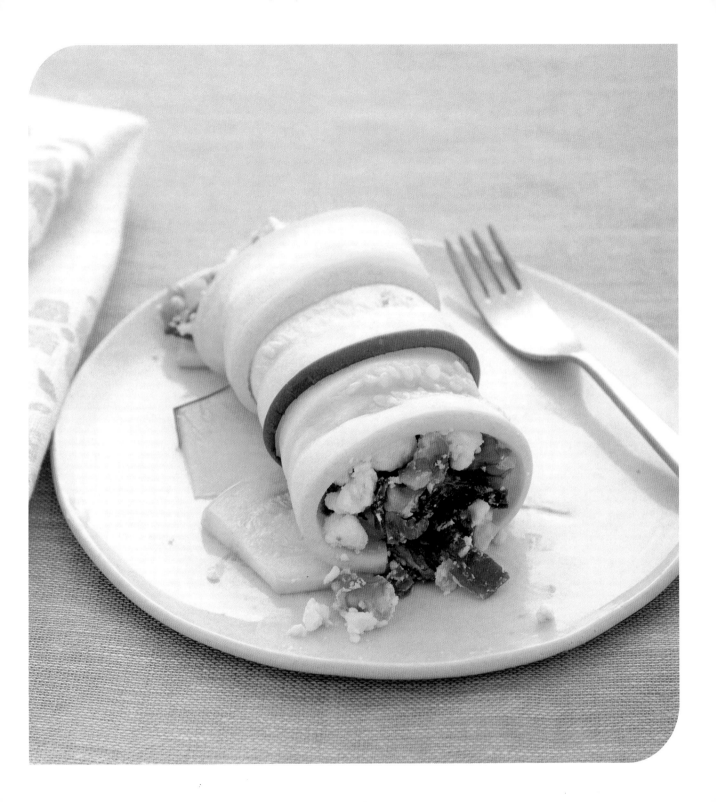

Tuscan Bean Wraps

In Tuscany, beans are just as popular as pasta. Here, the combination of smooth white bean puree, warm tortillas, savory tomato dressing, and Parmesan is mouthwatering, to say the least. Cut the rolls into slices for a great party appetizer. You can also use the pureed beans as a dip with fennel, endive, radicchio, jicama, or other crunchy veggies.

2 plum tomatoes, chopped

8 large black olives, pitted and minced

2 tablespoons minced shallots

2 teaspoons balsamic vinegar

1/4 teaspoon fresh lemon juice

Freshly ground black pepper

1 can (15 1/2 ounces) cannellini beans, rinsed and drained

2 garlic cloves

2 tablespoons extra-virgin olive oil

2 tablespoons 0% plain Greek yogurt

1 teaspoon dried oregano

4 whole wheat tortillas (8-inch)

1/4 cup grated Parmesan cheese

1 Preheat the oven to 425°F.

2 Combine the tomatoes, olives, shallots, vinegar, lemon juice, and pepper to taste in a bowl.

3 Put the beans, garlic, oil, yogurt, and oregano in a food processor and puree into a smooth spread.

4 Arrange the tortillas in a single layer on a baking sheet. Spread half of each tortilla with the bean puree. Spoon the tomato mixture on top and sprinkle on the Parmesan. Fold the tortillas in half. Bake for 3 to 5 minutes, or until the cheese melts. Serve hot.

PER SERVING: 305 calories (102 from fat), 10 g protein, 11 g fat (2 g saturated fat), 42 g carbohydrates, 7 g fiber, 4 mg cholesterol, 658 mg sodium

Black-Eyed Pea Wraps

Put a little Southern style into your day with black-eyed peas! Mixed with a colorful combination of cucumbers, red peppers, olives, and red onion, these tasty beans make a fresh, crunchy filling for a wrap. Not a fan of black-eyed peas? Black, pinto, kidney, or cannellini beans are perfect subsitutes. Add 2 or 3 whole grain crackers such as ak-mak, reduced-fat Triscuits, or Ry-Krisps to each serving. Orange and grapefruit segments tossed with some chopped mint make a refreshing dessert to finish it off.

3 tablespoons extra-virgin olive oil

2 tablespoons fresh lemon juice

2 teaspoons chopped fresh oregano or 1 teaspoon dried

Freshly ground black pepper

4 cups peeled and diced cucumbers (2 medium)

1 can (14 ounces) black-eyed peas, rinsed and drained

1/3 cup chopped roasted red peppers

2/3 cup diced fresh red bell pepper

1/2 cup crumbled fat-free feta cheese

1/2 cup finely chopped red onion

2 garlic cloves, minced

2 tablespoons chopped black olives

4 large romaine lettuce leaves, center ribs cut out

1 Whisk together the oil, lemon juice, oregano, and black pepper to taste in a large bowl.

2 Add the cucumbers, black-eyed peas, roasted peppers, fresh bell peppers, feta, onion, garlic, and olives to the bowl and toss well to coat all the ingredients.

3 Divide the salad among the lettuce leaves, roll up, and serve.

PER SERVING: 216 calories (103 from fat), 9 g protein, 11 g fat (2 g saturated fat), 19 g carbohydrates, 5 g fiber, 3 mg cholesterol, 425 mg sodium

Baked Falafel Wraps

These scrumptious Middle Eastern falafel patties are baked, not fried, which means you can enjoy them more often! While pita is the traditional wrapper, try lettuce leaves for a crispier and even skinnier version. Top with the tangy, super creamy Avocado-Yogurt Sauce or the to-die-for tzatziki (from the Chicken Tzatziki Wraps, page 100).

4 scallions, chopped

½ cup diced mushrooms

2 cans (15 ounces each) chickpeas, not drained

6 garlic cloves, coarsely chopped

½ cup chopped onion

3 tablespoons chopped cilantro

1 tablespoon chopped parsley

1 tablespoon curry powder

1 teaspoon ground cumin

1 cup dried whole wheat bread crumbs

3 egg whites, lightly beaten

4 large romaine lettuce leaves, center ribs cut out

Avocado-Yogurt Sauce (recipe follows)

1 Preheat the oven to 350°F.

2 Heat a skillet over medium heat. Coat with cooking spray. Add the scallions and mushrooms and cook until the mushrooms are reduced by half and the scallions are browned and softened, 5 to 8 minutes. Turn off the heat and let stand for a minute or two.

3 Put the chickpeas and their liquid in a food processor along with the garlic and onion. Blend until the mixture is creamy. Transfer the chickpea mixture to a bowl and stir in the cilantro, parsley, curry powder, and cumin. Then add the bread crumbs and egg whites, followed by the cooked mushroom mixture.

4 Coat a baking sheet with cooking spray. Using moist hands, shape a heaping tablespoon of the mixture into a ball and place on the baking sheet. Continue until all the mixture is used, leaving a 1-inch space between the balls. With the palm of your hand, gently flatten each ball.

5 Bake for 20 minutes, or until golden brown. Serve warm rolled in a romaine leaf with Avocado-Yogurt Sauce.

PER SERVING: 247 calories (54 from fat), 14 g protein, 6 g fat (0.5 g saturated fat), 37 g carbohydrates, 10 g fiber, 0 mg cholesterol, 287 mg sodium

AVOCADO-YOGURT SAUCE

MAKES ABOUT 4 CUPS

A perfect topper for the Baked Falafel Wraps, this lemony sauce is also fabulous on chicken, fish, or other vegetables. I'm a huge fan of nonfat Greek yogurt because it's good for your bones, your blood pressure, and your immune system. Use it instead of sour cream on baked potatoes, and blend it with different herbs to make other yummy dips.

2 large Hass avocados

1 cup seeded and chopped cucumber

4 garlic cloves, coarsely chopped

½ cup 0% plain Greek yogurt

1 cup fresh lemon juice

¼ teaspoon crushed red pepper flakes

2 tablespoons chopped cilantro

2 tablespoons chopped mint

1 Scoop the avocado flesh into a food processor. Add the cucumber, garlic, yogurt, and lemon juice and blend until smooth. Pour into a bowl and stir in the pepper flakes, cilantro, and mint.

2 Chill for at least 1 hour before serving. The sauce will keep in the refrigerator for 2 days.

PER SERVING (1 cup): 154 calories (95 from fat), 5 g protein, 4 g fat (1 g saturated fat), 14 g carbohydrates, 5 g fiber, 0 mg cholesterol, 19 mg sodium

Eat More to Lose More?

Eating small, frequent meals is the key to keeping your metabolism revved up all day, constantly burning what you consume. Eat four to six small meals and two to three light snacks. Remember to stretch, exercise, and eat healthy, because every bite of food you take requires your body to break it down. This way of eating ensures that your body has energy to burn throughout the day. And if you're not hungry, you won't give in to eating high-calorie, high-fat snacks.

Can't Beet
These Wraps

You can't find a veggie sweeter—or a prettier shade of violet—than beets, and they make for a fantastic wrap filler! For convenience, purchase some that are already peeled, steamed, and ready to eat. (You'll find them in the produce section.) Combine beets with asparagus and you've got a super colorful, knockout lunch or dinner!

¼ cup chopped walnuts

1 tablespoon extra-virgin olive oil

20 asparagus spears, cut into 1-inch pieces

Freshly ground black pepper

1 package (8 ounces) peeled and ready-to-eat steamed beets, cut into large dice

¼ cup nonfat plain yogurt

¼ cup crumbled fat-free feta cheese

2 tablespoons chopped chives

2 cups mixed greens

4 vegetable tortillas (8-inch), warmed

1 Place the walnuts in a skillet over medium-high heat. Shake the nuts continuously until they start to turn color, 3 to 5 minutes. Remove immediately from the heat and set aside.

2 Heat the oil in a medium to large skillet over medium-high heat. Add the asparagus and cook for 5 to 7 minutes. Season with black pepper to taste and transfer to a bowl.

3 Add the beets, nuts, yogurt, feta, chives, and greens to the bowl and toss well.

4 Spread one-quarter of the beet mixture in the middle of each tortilla, leaving a ½-inch border on the sides and bottom. Fold the bottom end of the tortilla up and over the filling, fold in both sides, and continue rolling. Serve.

PER SERVING: 223 calories (95 from fat), 12 g protein, 11 g fat (1 g saturated fat), 23 g carbohydrates, 6 g fiber, 2 mg cholesterol, 326 mg sodium

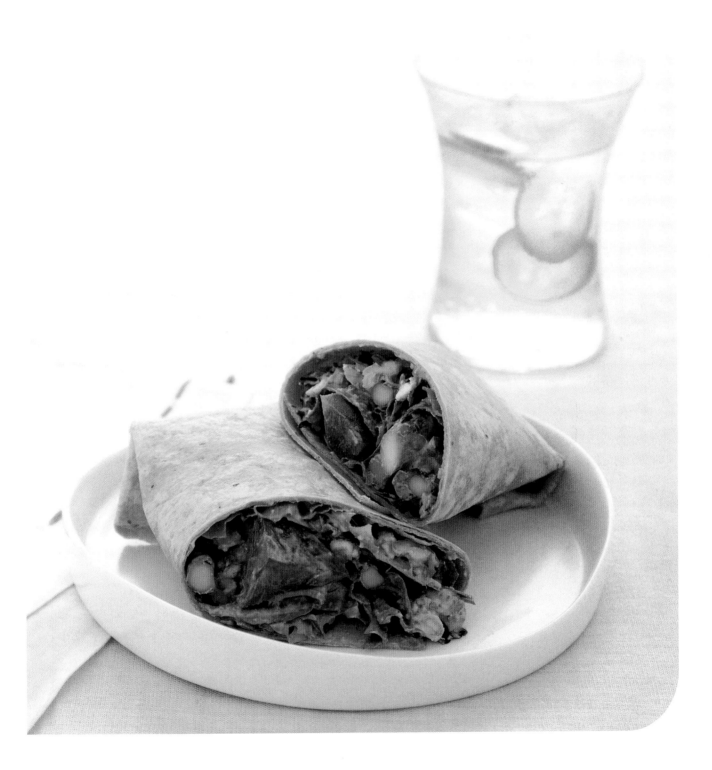

Fruit *and* Cheese Wraps

Take the classic fruit and cheese platter concept on the road with these Granny Smith and goat cheese wraps. Think outside the wrap and use pears or in-season peaches instead of apples, arugula in place of the spinach, or pecans or almonds instead of walnuts. Any combination will win you and your taste buds over.

1/3 cup chopped walnuts

4 cups baby spinach leaves

1 Granny Smith apple, sliced

5 ounces fresh goat cheese, crumbled

2 tablespoons apple cider vinegar

2 tablespoons maple syrup

2 tablespoons extra-virgin olive oil

4 spinach-flavored whole wheat tortillas (8-inch)

1 Place the walnuts in a skillet over medium-high heat. Shake the nuts continuously until they start to turn color, 3 to 5 minutes. Remove immediately from the heat and transfer to a large bowl.

2 Add the spinach, apple, and cheese to the bowl and toss lightly.

3 Whisk together the vinegar, maple syrup, and oil in a small bowl.

4 Spoon one-quarter of the salad onto each tortilla, leaving a 1/2-inch border on the sides and bottom. Drizzle the dressing on top. Fold the bottom end of the tortilla up and over the filling, fold in both sides, and continue rolling. Serve.

PER SERVING: 391 calories (199 from fat), 13 g protein, 22 g fat (7 g saturated fat), 38 g carbohydrates, 5 g fiber, 16 mg cholesterol, 502 mg sodium

Greek Salad Wraps Hollywood-Style

Adding creamy avocado, strawberries, and spinach puts an exotic twist on a classic Greek salad. If fresh strawberries aren't in season, buy them frozen and thaw before mixing in. And no need to limit this wrap to the summer months; in the winter, try juicy sliced pears and apples, and in the spring, chop up some crunchy asparagus.

⅓ cup extra-virgin olive oil

3 tablespoons fresh lemon juice

1½ teaspoons dried oregano

Pinch of crushed red pepper flakes

1 Hass avocado, cut into ½ -inch cubes

6 plum tomatoes, cut into ½-inch cubes

1 cucumber, peeled and cut into ½-inch cubes

3 cups (packed) chopped spinach leaves

2 cups sliced strawberries

½ cup crumbled fat-free feta cheese

Freshly ground black pepper

4 whole wheat tortillas (8-inch), spinach-flavored or plain, warmed

1 Whisk the oil, lemon juice, oregano, and pepper flakes together in a small bowl. Set aside.

2 Combine the avocado, tomatoes, cucumber, spinach, strawberries, and feta in a large bowl. Season with some black pepper. Toss the salad with the dressing.

3 Spread one-quarter of the salad in the middle of each tortilla, leaving a ½-inch border on the sides and bottom. Fold the bottom end of the tortilla up and over the filling, fold in both sides, and continue rolling. Serve.

PER SERVING: 437 calories (235 from fat), 12 g protein, 26 g fat (3 g saturated fat), 43 g carbohydrates, 9 g fiber, 3 mg cholesterol, 532 mg sodium

Brie and Fruit Wraps *with* Parsley Pesto

Fruit and cheese strike again! This wrap is filled with pears and cranberries paired with Parmesan, Brie, and zesty pesto. Although pesto is traditionally made with basil, it can also be whipped up with parsley (which this recipe calls for), spinach, arugula, or cilantro. Feel free to replace the dried cranberries with raisins, currants, or chopped apricots.

1½ cups loosely packed parsley leaves

3 tablespoons tarragon leaves

2 garlic cloves

½ cup grated Parmesan cheese

¼ cup extra-virgin olive oil

4 whole wheat tortillas (8-inch)

3 pears, cut lengthwise into thin wedges

¼ cup dried cranberries

10 ounces light Brie cheese

1 cup mixed greens

1 Combine the parsley, tarragon, garlic, and Parmesan in the food processor. Pulse several times to chop the mixture. With the machine running, slowly add the oil and process until pureed. Scrape the pesto into a bowl and set aside.

2 Preheat the oven to 350°F.

3 Arrange the tortillas in a single layer on a baking sheet. Spread 1 tablespoon of the pesto on the tortillas, then layer on the pears and cranberries, and top with the cheese.

4 Bake for 3 to 5 minutes, until the cheese begins to melt. Remove from the oven, and top with the greens. Fold the bottom end of the tortilla up and over the filling, fold in both sides, and continue rolling. Serve hot.

PER SERVING: 500 calories (195 from fat), 25 g protein, 22 g fat (8 g saturated fat), 57 g carbohydrates, 8 g fiber, 42 mg cholesterol, 1,000 mg sodium

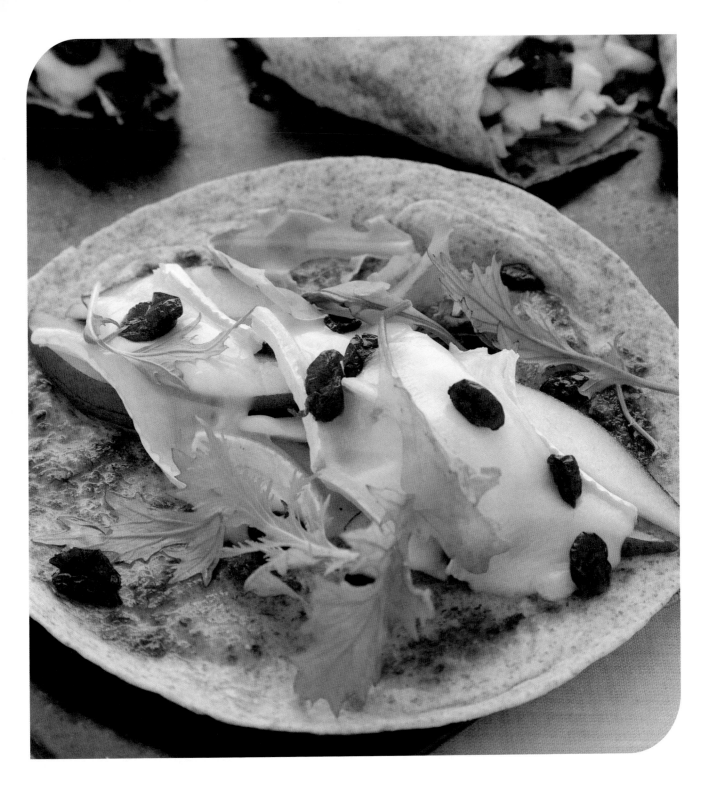

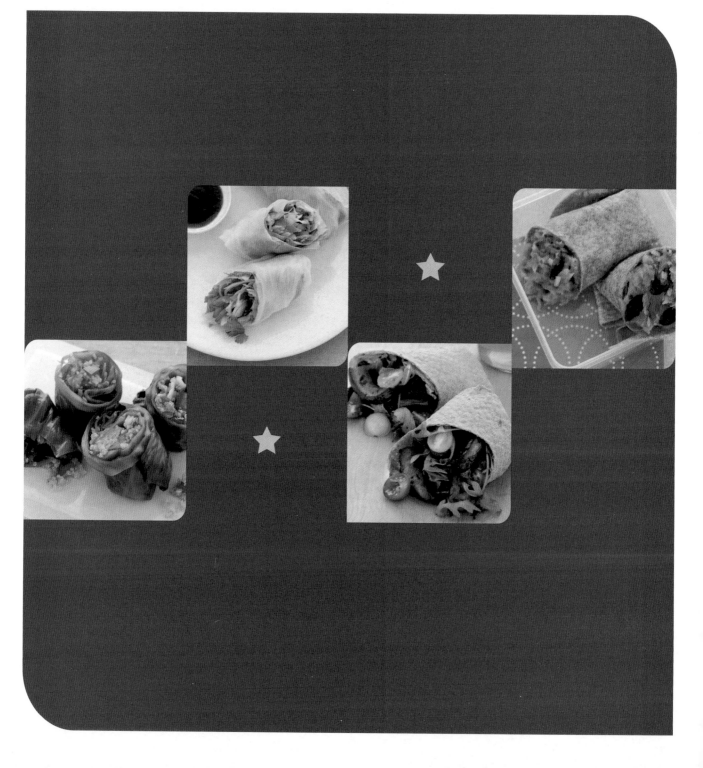

★ Vegan Wraps

Veganism is growing by leaps and bounds, with many people making the change to this lifestyle. Vegans eat no animal products for health reasons as well as out of concern for the way animals are bred, raised, and slaughtered. They eat no meat, no fish, no chicken, no dairy, no eggs, and no honey. Documented benefits of a pure vegan lifestyle include permanent weight reduction, healthy blood pressure, low serum cholesterol, and low blood sugar numbers as well as risk reduction for cardiovascular disease and other diet-related illnesses. Some who suffer from migraines and allergies have found relief eating a vegan diet, too.

If you're interested in finding out more about becoming a vegan, there's a world of information available at your bookstore or library and on the Internet. But even if you're not ready to forgo animal products entirely, I promise you will love these winning vegan wraps on their own merits and never miss the meat, eggs, or dairy for an instant.

Summer Rolls

Vietnamese summer rolls make colorful, crowd-pleasing appetizers. Fill them up with pork, shrimp, rice, vermicelli, or, as this recipe calls for, veggies and herbs. Lay all your ingredients out beforehand and whip up a dipping sauce with a combination of Sriracha and ponzu sauces, both available in Asian markets or in the international aisle of many supermarkets. Summer rolls are best when freshly made, but they can be prepared several hours ahead. Cover them with damp paper towels and plastic wrap and refrigerate until ready to serve accompanied by the dipping sauce.

¼ **cup Sriracha chili sauce**

¼ **cup ponzu sauce**

8 **rice papers**

8 **Bibb lettuce leaves**

1 **carrot, shredded**

1 **red bell pepper, very thinly sliced**

2 **scallions, thinly sliced**

16 **mint leaves**

16 **cilantro sprigs**

1 Whisk together the Sriracha and ponzu sauces in a bowl. Set aside.

2 Put some water in a shallow dish large enough to hold one rice paper. Immerse one wrapper in the water and let it soak just until softened, 5 to 15 seconds. Remove the rice paper from the water, put it on a clean kitchen towel, and let sit for 20 to 30 seconds so the excess water is absorbed.

3 Layer the lettuce, carrot, bell pepper, scallions, mint, and cilantro in the center of each rice paper. Fold the bottom end of the rice paper up and over the filling, fold in both sides, and continue rolling. Serve.

PER SERVING (2 rolls): 104 calories (6 from fat), 4 g protein, 0.5 g fat (0 g saturated fat), 22 g carbohydrates, 2 g fiber, 0 mg cholesterol, 382 mg sodium

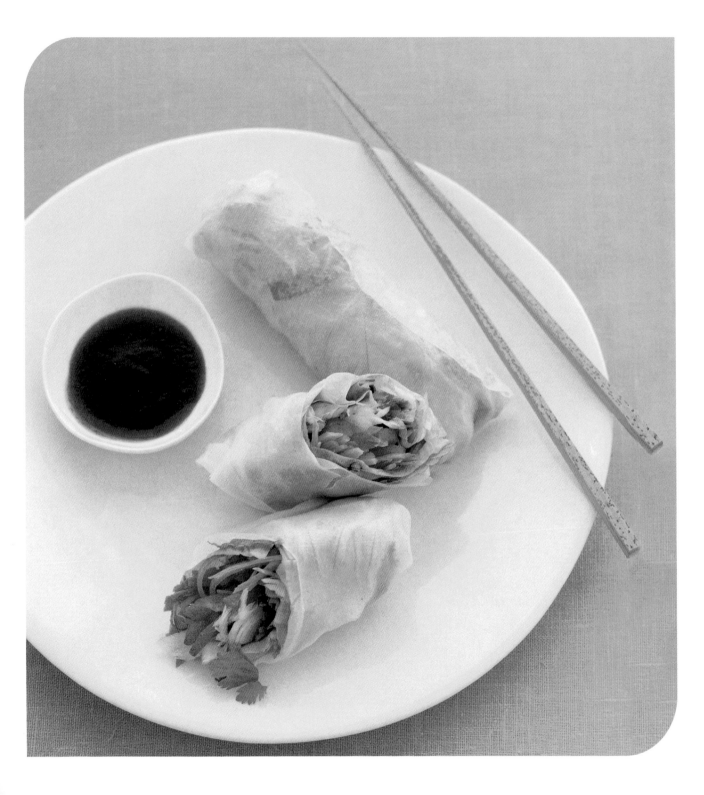

Tofu Sloppy Joe Wraps

★ :: **MAKES 4**

Traditional Sloppy Joes are made with ground beef, but you and your Hollywood bod will love this low-fat, low-cal version made with high-protein tofu. Try Muir Glen Organic Tomato Ketchup to mix in.

²/₃ cup ketchup

1 tablespoon maple syrup

1 teaspoon Dijon mustard

½ teaspoon chili powder

¼ teaspoon ground cumin

2 tablespoons extra-virgin olive oil

2 garlic cloves, minced

1 small onion, diced

1 red bell pepper, chopped

1 pound extra-firm tofu, diced

2½ tablespoons low-sodium soy sauce

4 whole wheat tortillas (8-inch), sun-dried tomato–flavored or plain, warmed

1 Whisk together the ketchup, maple syrup, mustard, chili powder, and cumin in a small bowl. Set aside.

2 Heat the oil in a skillet over medium heat. Add the garlic, onion, and bell pepper. Cook until the vegetables are soft, 6 to 8 minutes.

3 Turn the heat down to low. Add the tofu and soy sauce and cook until the tofu begins to get crisp, about 8 minutes. Stir in the ketchup mixture and fold thoroughly until all of the tofu is covered with the ketchup mixture.

4 Spread one-quarter of the filling in the middle of each tortilla, leaving a ½-inch border on the sides and bottom. Fold the bottom end of the tortilla up and over the filling, fold in both sides, and continue rolling. Serve hot.

PER SERVING: 382 calories (132 from fat), 17 g protein, 15 g fat (2 g saturated fat), 48 g carbohydrates, 6 g fiber, 0 mg cholesterol, 1,146 mg sodium

Tofu Puppy Wraps

★ :: **MAKES 4**

Soy hot dogs are a tasty and nutritious quick fix. Check the package for sodium content as some brands contain a lot more than others.

8 soy hot dogs

4 whole wheat tortillas (8-inch)

2 teaspoons Dijon mustard

1 ounce sliced Swiss-style soy cheese

½ cup shredded soy Cheddar cheese

1 Preheat the oven to 350°F.

2 Heat a ridged grill pan over medium-high heat. Add the hot dogs and cook, turning occasionally, until they are marked on all sides, 3 to 5 minutes.

3 Arrange the tortillas on a baking sheet. Spread ½ teaspoon mustard and put 2 hot dogs on each tortilla and top with the cheeses. Roll up and bake for 3 to 5 minutes. Serve immediately.

PER SERVING: 260 calories (33 from fat), 26 g protein, 4 g fat (0 g saturated fat), 30 g carbohydrates, 4 g fiber, 0 mg cholesterol, 928 mg sodium

Red Carpet Treadmill Routine

Kelly Preston hated the treadmill. Just walking for 20 minutes was boring for this multitasking jet-setter until I introduced her to a treadmill routine that kept her workout interesting—and the pounds off! Here's the secret: Vary the incline. Set your treadmill to raise the incline 1 percent every minute for 10 minutes, then lower the incline 1 percent every minute for another 10 minutes. You'll break a sweat and get your heart rate up way before boredom sets in.

Make sure to walk softly to protect your joints, and cool down afterward.

Want to work your booty harder? Squeeze your glutes every time your foot moves to the back of the treadmill. You'll see some definition in no time!

Spicy Tofu Lettuce Wraps

★ :: **MAKES 8**

Ginger, spicy mustard, and cilantro give this tofu wrap a lively kick. Good lettuce wraps are all about the contrast of warm, flavorful fillings and the cool crunch of the outside, so feel free to make them with your favorite burrito or taco stuffers. If you are serving these tofu wraps at home, pass the filling and lettuce leaves separately so each person can make his or her own wrap. Serve a brisk salad of cucumbers, scallions, and rice vinegar alongside.

¼ cup low-sodium soy sauce

2 teaspoons chopped cilantro

1 teaspoon minced garlic

1 teaspoon grated fresh ginger

1 teaspoon toasted sesame seeds

1 teaspoon spicy mustard

1 teaspoon hoisin sauce

½ teaspoon maple syrup

1 pound extra-firm tofu, cut crosswise in ½-inch slices

2 teaspoons extra-virgin olive oil

8 iceberg lettuce cups

½ onion, thinly sliced

1 cup alfalfa sprouts

2 tablespoons slivered almonds, toasted

1 Whisk together the soy sauce, cilantro, garlic, ginger, sesame seeds, mustard, hoisin sauce, and maple syrup in a shallow dish large enough to hold the tofu in a single layer.

2 Add the tofu to the marinade, turning to coat, and refrigerate for 30 minutes to 1 hour.

3 Heat the oil in a skillet over medium heat. Add the tofu and marinade and cook, turning the tofu once with a spatula, until the tofu is hot and the marinade is reduced and thickened. Divide the tofu and sauce among the lettuce leaves.

4 Top with the onion, sprouts, and almonds. Roll up and serve.

PER SERVING (2 wraps): 187 calories (93 from fat), 14 g protein, 10 g fat (1.3 g saturated fat), 9 g carbohydrates, 3 g fiber, 0 mg cholesterol, 626 mg sodium

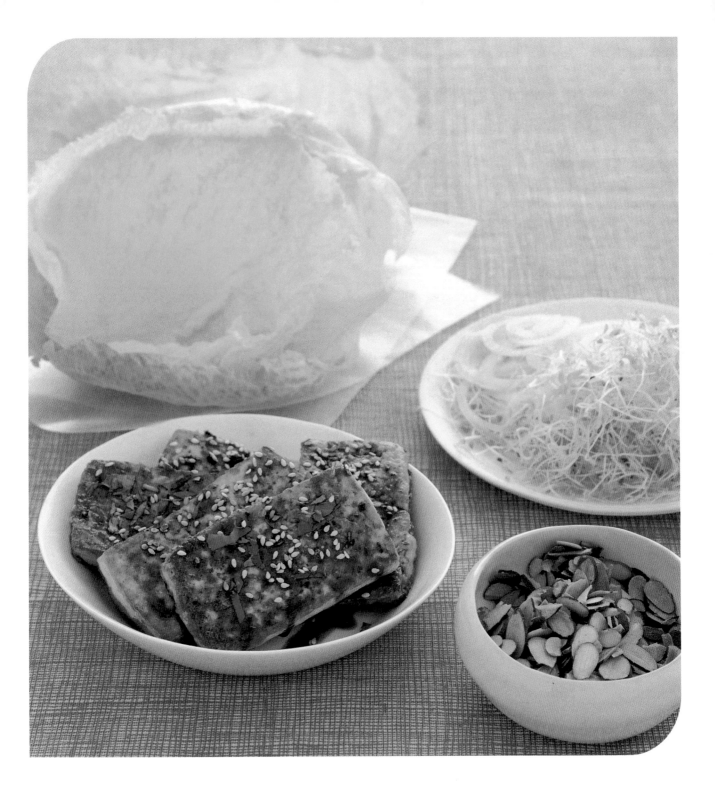

Tofu-Tapenade Wraps

Tofu is usually paired with Asian ingredients, but this dish heads to the South of France. Tapenade, a classic Provençal olive paste, gives the tofu a vibrant Mediterranean flavor. Keep extra tapenade on hand to use as a spread for meats or a dip for vegetables.

¼ cup chopped pitted green olives

¼ cup chopped pitted kalamata olives

1 teaspoon grated lemon zest

1 teaspoon extra-virgin olive oil

2 tablespoons fresh lemon juice

1 tablespoon red wine vinegar

1 tablespoon honey

2 teaspoons Dijon mustard

1 garlic clove, minced

1 teaspoon chopped rosemary

1½ cups sliced red onions

½ cup sliced mushrooms

3 tablespoons balsamic vinegar

1 pound extra-firm tofu, cut crosswise into ½-inch slices

4 garlic-flavored whole wheat tortillas (8-inch), warmed

1 Combine the olives, lemon zest, and oil in a food processor. Pulse until finely chopped but don't puree to a paste. Set the tapenade aside (or refrigerate for up to 1 week).

2 Combine the lemon juice, red wine vinegar, honey, mustard, garlic, and rosemary in a small bowl. Mix well.

3 Coat a skillet with cooking spray and heat over medium heat. Add the onions and mushrooms and cook, stirring occasionally, until lightly browned. Remove to a bowl and stir in the balsamic vinegar. Wipe out the skillet.

4 Coat the same skillet with more cooking spray and heat over low heat. Add the tofu in a single layer and cook until browned, 4 to 5 minutes. Use a spatula to turn the tofu and cook on the other side until browned. Add the lemon juice mixture and cook until the sauce thickens, 5 to 6 minutes.

5 Smear the tortillas evenly with the tapenade and top with the tofu and onion-mushroom mixture. Fold the bottom end of the tortilla up and over the filling, fold in both sides, and continue rolling. Serve.

PER SERVING: 321 calories (93 from fat), 16 g protein, 10 g fat (1 g saturated fat), 42 g carbohydrates, 5 g fiber, 0 mg cholesterol, 504 mg sodium

Ratatouille Wraps *with* Pistachio Pesto

If your plate of veggies is bursting with color, chances are that it's also bursting with essential vitamins and antioxidants. This ratatouille is fantastic in a wrap, but mix it up by spooning it into hollowed-out zucchini cups or red pepper wedges. Double the recipe and you'll have enough to spoon over whole wheat pasta.

1 cup basil leaves

$\frac{1}{4}$ cup shelled pistachios

4 whole garlic cloves + 2 garlic cloves, minced

$\frac{1}{2}$ cup + 4 teaspoons + 1 tablespoon extra-virgin olive oil

1 medium eggplant, cut crosswise into 8 thin slices

$\frac{1}{2}$ onion, diced

2 yellow summer squash, chopped

1 zucchini, chopped

2 plum tomatoes, chopped

2 tablespoons chopped parsley

4 whole wheat tortillas (8-inch), warmed

1. Combine the basil, pistachios, and whole garlic cloves in a food processor. Pulse several times to chop the mixture. With the machine running, slowly add $\frac{1}{2}$ cup of the oil and process until pureed.

2. Heat 2 teaspoons of the oil in a skillet over medium heat. Add 4 slices of the eggplant (don't crowd the pan) and cook for 3 to 5 minutes per side until browned and tender. Remove to paper towels to drain. Repeat with the remaining eggplant and additional oil as needed.

3. Heat the remaining 1 tablespoon oil in the skillet. Add the onion, squash, zucchini, tomatoes, and minced garlic. Cook until the vegetables are lightly browned, 3 to 4 minutes. Stir in the parsley.

4. Place 2 eggplant slices on each tortilla. Top with one-quarter of the squash mixture and 2 tablespoons of the pesto. Fold the bottom end of the tortilla up and over the filling, fold in both sides, and continue rolling.

PER SERVING: 570 calories (378 from fat), 10 g protein, 42 g fat (5.7 g saturated fat), 45 g carbohydrates, 11 g fiber, 0 mg cholesterol, 344 mg sodium

Confetti Quinoa *and* Cabbage Wraps

While its spelling might trip you up, crunchy quinoa is the grain of all grains: It's packed with protein. Rinse well before cooking (to remove the bitter coating of saponins), cook, and then mix with a blend of colorful chopped veggies for a wrap filling that looks just like confetti.

¼ cup quinoa

3 tablespoons fresh lemon juice

5 teaspoons extra-virgin olive oil

½ teaspoon Dijon mustard

1 teaspoon chopped fresh dill

3 plum tomatoes, chopped

1 Hass avocado, sliced

1 cucumber, peeled, seeded, and chopped

1 carrot, grated

8 red cabbage leaves

1 Put the quinoa in a fine-mesh strainer and rinse under running water until it no longer looks soapy.

2 Bring ½ cup water to a boil in a small saucepan. Add the quinoa, cover, and simmer for 15 minutes, or until the water is absorbed. When done, it should be light and fluffy when tossed with a fork. Set aside to cool, then transfer to a bowl. Add the tomatoes, avocado, cucumber, and carrot.

3 In a small bowl, stir together the lemon juice, oil, mustard, and dill. Pour over the quinoa and toss well.

4 Bring a large pot of water to a boil. Fill a bowl with ice and water. Add the cabbage leaves to the boiling water and cook until the leaves are pliable, 30 seconds to 1 minute. Using tongs, transfer the leaves to the ice water to cool. Drain well and pat dry.

5 Fill each leaf with the quinoa mixture, roll up, and serve.

PER SERVING (2 wraps): 187 calories (108 from fat), 4 g protein, 12 g fat (2 g saturated fat), 19 g carbohydrates, 5 g fiber, 0 mg cholesterol, 45 mg sodium

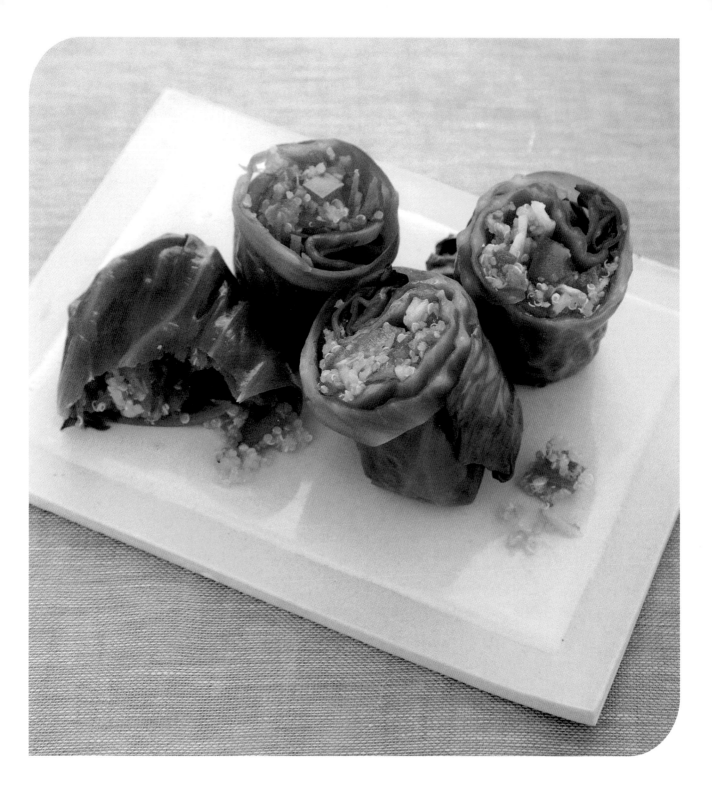

Quinoa Wraps

I love this protein powerhouse grain so much that I've included two recipes for it. When you cook it, quinoa becomes light and fluffy—a perfect wrap stuffer. Get crafty with your own salads or wrap fillings by adding diced and blanched vegetables, toasted nuts and seeds, and herbs and spices of your choice.

½ cup quinoa

1 can (15 ounces) chickpeas, rinsed and drained

½ cup dried cranberries

½ cup raisins

¼ cup sunflower seeds

2 tablespoons chopped parsley

¼ cup extra-virgin olive oil

Juice of ½ lemon

1 teaspoon Dijon mustard

1 tablespoon chopped fresh dill

4 whole wheat tortillas (8-inch)

1 Put the quinoa in a fine-mesh strainer and rinse under running water until it no longer looks soapy.

2 Bring 1 cup water to a boil in a medium saucepan. Add the quinoa, cover, and simmer for 15 minutes, or until the water is absorbed. When done, it should be light and fluffy when tossed with a fork. Set aside to cool.

3 Add the chickpeas, cranberries, raisins, sunflower seeds, and parsley to the quinoa and mix well.

4 Whisk together the oil, lemon juice, mustard, and dill in a small bowl.

5 Spread one-quarter of the quinoa mixture in the center of each tortilla, leaving a ½-inch border on the sides and bottom. Drizzle on the dressing. Fold the bottom end of the tortilla up and over the filling, fold in both sides, and continue rolling. Serve.

PER SERVING: 587 calories (202 from fat), 14 g protein, 22 g fat (3 g saturated fat), 88 g carbohydrates, 10 g fiber, 0 mg cholesterol, 609 mg sodium

Veggie Burger Wraps

I'm a big fan of frozen veggie burgers, but beware: They are not all created equal. Many are made with fillers, preservatives, and additives—none of which were grown in a garden. When reading labels, real vegetables like zucchini, carrots, and onions should be listed first. Also check for whopping sodium contents. Some of my favorites are made by Trader Joe's, Vitasoy, Dr. Praeger's, Amy's American, and Vivera. If you prefer your burgers hot and spicy, then add the jalapeño seeds to this veggie-licious wrap.

1½ teaspoons extra-virgin olive oil

1 cup sliced mushrooms

1 small sweet Maui onion, sliced

1 jalapeño pepper, minced and seeded

2 veggie burgers

4 whole wheat tortillas (8-inch), warmed

1 cup shredded Monterey Jack–style soy cheese

Spicy Ketchup (optional)

¼ cup ketchup

1 teaspoon ground white pepper

1 teaspoon chili powder

1 Heat the oil in a skillet over medium-high heat. Add the mushrooms, onion, and jalapeño. Cook until the vegetables are soft, 6 to 8 minutes. Transfer to a large bowl and set aside.

2 Add the veggie burgers to the same skillet and cook until heated through, 4 to 5 minutes on each side. Cut the burgers in half.

3 Place a half burger on each tortilla and top with the mushroom mixture and cheese. If using spicy ketchup, combine all ingredients in a bowl and top the burger with 1 tablespoon. Fold the bottom end of the tortilla up and over the filling, fold in both sides, and continue rolling. Serve.

PER SERVING: 285 calories (69 from fat), 17 g protein, 8 g fat (4 g saturated fat), 38 g carbohydrates, 5 g fiber, 1 mg cholesterol, 1,063 mg sodium

Sautéed Portobello Wraps

You can grill or broil thick, meaty portobello mushroom caps just like you would a hamburger, and you'll save yourself 400 calories! The portobellos in this wrap are sautéed with onions and paired with crunchy veggies. You can also try filling the caps with chopped vegetables and baking them with a sprinkle of Parmesan.

2 tablespoons chopped sun-dried (not oil-packed) tomatoes

1½ tablespoons red wine vinegar

1 teaspoon Dijon mustard

3 tablespoons + 1 teaspoon extra-virgin olive oil

3 large portobello mushrooms, cut into ½-inch-wide strips

½ onion, thinly sliced

1 cup halved cherry tomatoes

1 cup arugula

4 pieces (8 x 8-inch) whole wheat lavash

1 Whisk together the sun-dried tomatoes, vinegar, mustard, and 3 tablespoons of the oil in a small bowl. Set aside.

2 Heat the remaining 1 teaspoon oil in a skillet over medium-high heat. Add the mushrooms and onion and cook until softened and beginning to brown, 10 to 12 minutes.

3 Combine the sun-dried tomato dressing, sautéed vegetables, cherry tomatoes, and arugula in a large bowl. Fold together until all of the ingredients are coated with the dressing.

4 Spread one-quarter of the filling in the middle of each piece of lavash, roll up, and serve.

PER SERVING: 236 calories (125 from fat), 5 g protein, 14 g fat (2 g saturated fat), 27 g carbohydrates, 5 g fiber, 0 mg cholesterol, 104 mg sodium

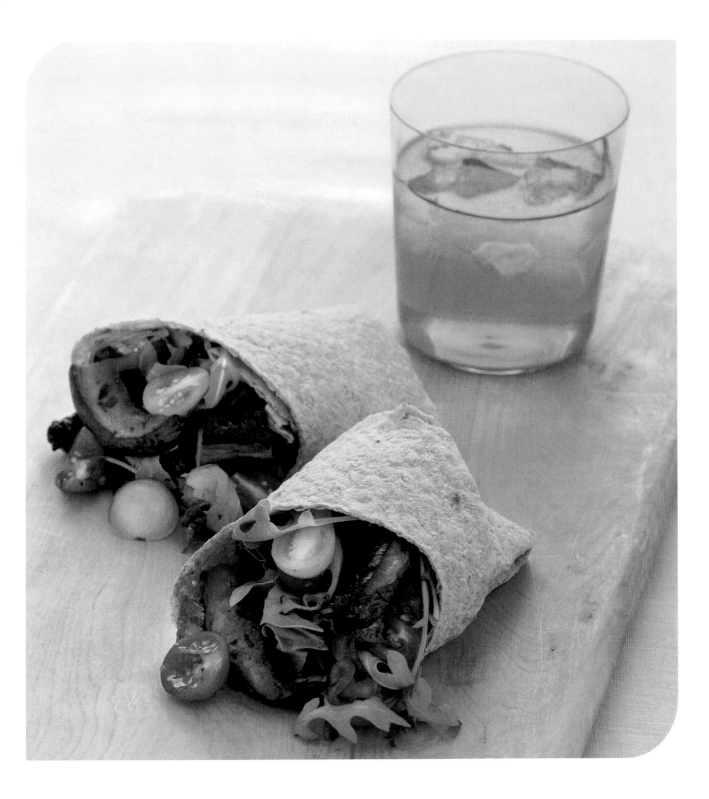

Mushroom-Tempeh Melt

Tempeh is a go-to vegan soy product with a nuttier flavor and chewier consistency than tofu. Tempeh can be marinated and then grilled, baked, or sautéed, as below. Mix it with some veggies and you'll have a heart-healthy, flavor-packed wrap filling that you can always count on.

1 tablespoon extra-virgin olive oil

12 ounces white mushrooms, sliced (about 1½ cups)

2 garlic cloves, minced

1 small red onion, sliced

½ cup diced red bell pepper

Freshly ground black pepper

½ cup dry red wine

1 teaspoon balsamic vinegar

1 package (8 ounces) tempeh, cut into 4 pieces

2 ounces shredded Swiss soy cheese

4 multigrain tortillas (8-inch), warmed

1 Heat the oil in a skillet over medium heat. Add the mushrooms and garlic and cook until the mushrooms give up their juices and the juices have mostly evaporated.

2 Add the onion, bell pepper, and black pepper to taste. Cook, stirring occasionally, until the mushrooms are browned and softened, about 10 minutes.

3 Reduce the heat to low and stir in the wine and vinegar. Add the tempeh and cook until the wine has evaporated, 4 to 6 minutes.

4 Remove the skillet from the heat. Sprinkle the cheese over the mushrooms and tempeh, cover the skillet, and set aside for a few minutes until the cheese is melted.

5 Spread one-quarter of the tempeh-mushroom mixture on each tortilla, leaving a ½-inch border on the sides and bottom. Fold the bottom end of the tortilla up and over the filling, fold in both sides, and continue rolling. Serve.

PER SERVING: 377 calories (127 from fat), 22 g protein, 14 g fat (3 g saturated fat), 38 g carbohydrates, 10 g fiber, 0 mg cholesterol, 469 mg sodium

Santa Fe Rice *and* Beans Wraps

★ :: **MAKES 4**

Like barley and quinoa, rice takes on the flavors of whatever it's cooked with. The brown rice in this wrap goes great with a spicy blend of tomatoes, corn, black beans, and cilantro. You can tuck this Tex-Mex mixture into tortillas or serve it as a main course with a refreshing avocado, orange, and arugula salad.

1½ teaspoons tomato paste

1 teaspoon cayenne pepper

1 teaspoon smoked paprika

1 cup brown rice

2 plum tomatoes, diced

¼ large onion, diced

½ green bell pepper, diced

2 tablespoons frozen corn kernels, thawed

1 teaspoon minced garlic

1 tablespoon chopped cilantro

1 can (15 ounces) black beans, rinsed and drained

4 whole wheat tortillas (8-inch)

1 Whisk together 2 cups water, the tomato paste, cayenne, and paprika in a saucepan. Add the rice, bring to a boil, cover, reduce the heat, and simmer until all the water is absorbed, 20 to 30 minutes. Remove from the heat.

2 While the rice is cooking, mix together the tomatoes, onion, bell pepper, corn, garlic, and cilantro in a bowl. Set the salsa aside.

3 Stir the beans into the cooked rice until combined.

4 Spread one-quarter of the bean-rice mixture in the center of each tortilla, leaving a ½-inch border on the sides and bottom. Top with the salsa. Fold the bottom end of the tortilla up and over the filling, fold in both sides, and continue rolling. Serve.

PER SERVING: 387 calories (31 from fat), 13 g protein, 3 g fat (0.5 g saturated fat), 79 g carbohydrates, 10 g fiber, 0 mg cholesterol, 626 mg sodium

Sweet Potato Burritos

When picking potatoes, go for orange rather than white. Sweet potatoes are packed with vitamins—and the small portion used in this wrap will keep you full for hours! Bake a few extras and top them with nonfat yogurt and some steamed broccoli or asparagus for a luscious lunch.

1½ pounds sweet potatoes (about 4)

¼ cup extra-virgin olive oil

Juice of ½ lemon

1 teaspoon Dijon mustard

1 red onion, chopped

½ cup chopped cilantro

¼ cup dried cranberries

4 whole wheat tortillas (8-inch), warmed

1 Preheat the oven to 375°F. Pierce the sweet potatoes all over with a fork and place them on a baking sheet. Bake for 45 minutes to 1 hour, or until tender when pierced with a knife.

2 While the potatoes are baking, whisk together the oil, lemon juice, and mustard in a bowl. Set aside.

3 When the potatoes are cool enough to handle, cut them in half and scoop the flesh into a large bowl. Mash the potatoes and add the onion, cilantro, and cranberries. Whisk the dressing again and fold into the potato mixture.

4 Spread one-quarter of the filling in the middle of each tortilla, leaving a ½-inch border on the sides and bottom. Fold the bottom end of the tortilla up and over the filling, fold in both sides, and continue rolling. Serve warm.

PER SERVING: 422 calories (141 from fat), 7 g protein, 16 g fat (2 g saturated fat), 66 g carbohydrates, 8 g fiber, 0 mg cholesterol, 444 mg sodium

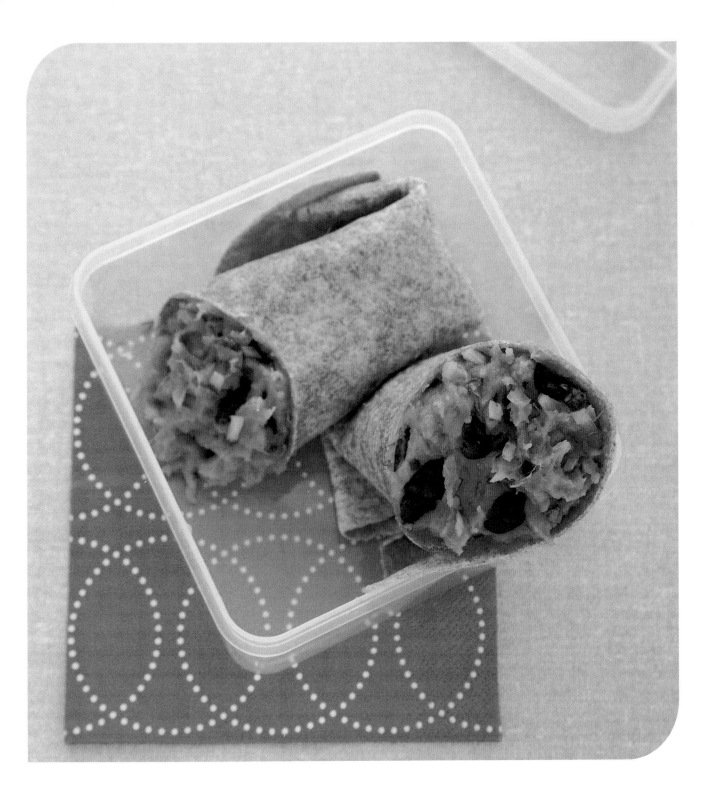

Hummus Wraps

Hummus, a delightful blend of cooked and mashed chickpeas, never fails as an appetizer, dip, or spread. Keep a bowl of hummus in the fridge all the time. Most people buy hummus, but it's just so easy—and super cheap—to make! Plus, you know exactly what goes into it. I've seen some pretty questionable varieties in the supermarket!

2 cups peeled, chopped cucumber

2 plum tomatoes, chopped (about 1 cup)

1 cup shredded carrots

1 cup alfalfa sprouts

²/₃ cup chopped roasted red peppers

²/₃ cup shredded Monterey Jack soy cheese

1 cup Hummus (recipe follows)

2 whole wheat pitas, split horizontally

1 Combine the cucumber, tomatoes, carrots, sprouts, roasted peppers, and cheese in a bowl. Stir in the hummus.

2 Spread one-quarter down the center of each pita half, roll up, and serve.

PER SERVING: 264 calories (14 from fat), 12 g protein, 14 g fat (5 g saturated fat), 27 g carbohydrates, 9 g fiber, 17 mg cholesterol, 423 mg sodium

24-Hour Prep for a Hot Love Scene

The day before your next hot date, drink a cup of 3 Ballerina Tea Dieters' Drink, which has a laxative effect. The day of your big scene, drink lots of water to hydrate the skin, so it glows, and eat no carbs at all, only lean protein and vegetables, so your tummy is extra flat.

HUMMUS

MAKES ABOUT 2 CUPS

1 can (15 ounces) chickpeas, rinsed and drained

½ large onion, chopped

3 garlic cloves, minced

2 tablespoons chopped cilantro

2 tablespoons chopped flat-leaf parsley

¼ cup extra-virgin olive oil

3 tablespoons fresh lemon juice + more to taste

1 tablespoon chopped fresh dill

½ teaspoon ground cumin

⅛ teaspoon cayenne pepper

Salt and freshly ground black pepper

1. Combine the chickpeas, onion, garlic, and 1 cup water in a saucepan. Bring to a simmer, cover, and cook for 8 minutes. Stir in the cilantro and parsley and let stand, uncovered, for 5 minutes.

2. Drain the chickpea mixture and transfer to a food processor. Add the oil, 3 tablespoons of lemon juice, the dill, cumin, and cayenne and process until smooth. Transfer to a bowl and cool to room temperature, stirring occasionally. Season with salt and black pepper and add lemon juice to taste.

3. Use immediately or store in a covered container in the refrigerator up to 5 days.

PER SERVING (¼ cup): 105 calories (69 from fat), 2 g protein, 8 g fat (1 g saturated fat), 8 g carbohydrates, 2 g fiber, 0 mg cholesterol, 64 mg sodium

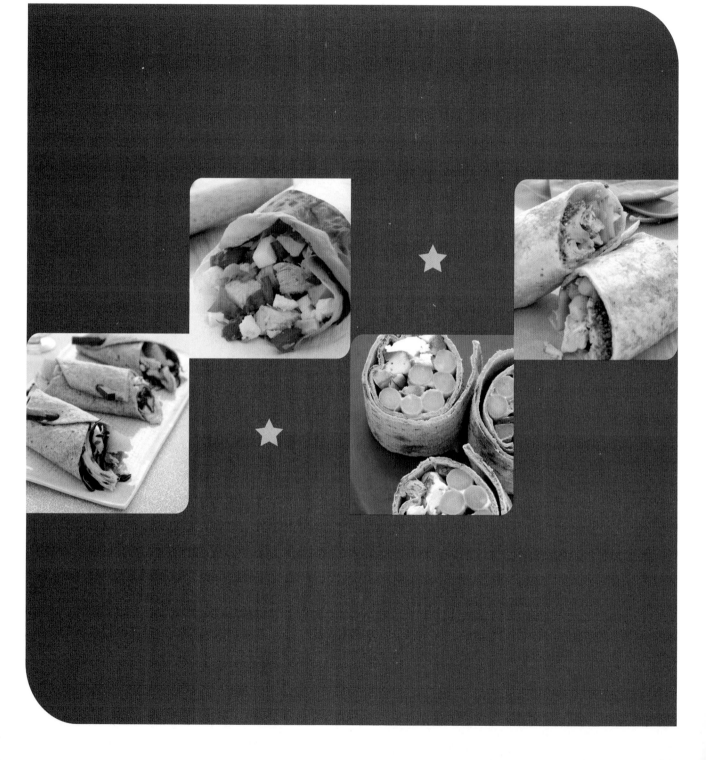

★ Chicken and Turkey Wraps

Delicious and versatile cooked chicken breasts provide the bulk of the protein in many of my most popular wraps. Please don't substitute processed chicken meat from the delicatessen; it's loaded with sodium and preservatives and should be avoided. Fortunately, it's incredibly easy to cook chicken breasts at home so you'll always have a lean, tasty, versatile protein on hand for your wrap creations.

There are a number of methods for preparing chicken breasts—baking, sautéing, grilling, poaching, and broiling all yield a delicious result, so just choose the one that suits you. For the sake of convenience, cook a few breasts at a time and refrigerate or freeze the extras. Before you get cooking, here are some tips to ensure juicy and flavorful chicken breasts every time.

★ **Be aware of portion size.** Start with boneless and skinless chicken breast halves that weigh about 6 ounces each.

★ **Watch out for added sodium.** Packaged chicken breasts are often plumped up with sodium and water. Look closely at the label; it should say "all-natural" or "no salt added." And aim for about 25 milligrams (the naturally present amount) of sodium per serving. Pre-marinated chicken may seem like an easy way to add a little zest and variety to your cooking, but they can easily contain as much as 500 milligrams of sodium per serving.

★ **Pound gently, cook evenly.** Most chicken breasts are thicker in the center, which makes them cook unevenly. You can remedy this easily by pounding the meat to an even thickness. Pounding takes no time at all, and it noticeably reduces the cooking time. Place the chicken breast between two sheets of plastic wrap on a cutting board. Using a flat meat pounder or rolling pin, lightly pound the breast until it is about 1/2 inch thick throughout. You just want to flatten the thickest part a bit, not beat holes in the meat! Remove the chicken from the plastic, season, and cook.

★ **Control temperature.** Chicken needs to be cooked to 170°F to kill potentially harmful bacteria, but a pounded breast is so thin that it is difficult, if not impossible, to get an accurate temperature reading with an instant-read meat thermometer. And because chicken breast is very lean, the meat can dry out quickly during cooking. Fortunately, overcooking is easy to avoid. Professional cooks often test boneless cuts like chicken breast (and steak) by touch. Press the chicken breast in the center with your fingertip. If it is underdone, it will still feel squishy and soft. If the chicken is cooked properly, it will bounce back. Or check for doneness by cutting a nick into the center of the chicken with the tip of a sharp knife— the meat should look opaque.

Let the chicken breast stand for about 5 minutes before slicing. This short wait allows the juices to settle and redistribute themselves. If you slice before the chicken has rested, the hot juices will run out, resulting in dry meat. After the chicken has cooled for a few minutes, it can be sliced or cut into chunks as the recipe requires.

★ **Store properly.** Cooked chicken breast can be cooled, covered, and refrigerated for a couple of days, or wrapped airtight and frozen for up to 2 months.

Waldorf Chicken Wraps

Chopped apple, celery, and walnuts add an agreeable crunch to this classic chicken salad. Balsamic vinegar is also a key ingredient: It's sweet, flavorful, and not too puckery. Serve the salad in lettuce leaves or warm tortillas.

4 boneless, skinless chicken breast halves (6 ounces each), cooked and cut into $1/2$-inch cubes

$1/2$ apple, chopped

$1/2$ cup chopped celery

2 scallions, chopped

$1/4$ cup chopped walnuts

3 tablespoons balsamic vinegar

$1/2$ cup fat-free mayonnaise

1 teaspoon Dijon mustard

Freshly ground black pepper

4 large butter lettuce leaves

1 Combine the chicken, apple, celery, scallions, and walnuts in a bowl. Set aside.

2 Mix the vinegar, mayonnaise, and mustard in a small bowl until thoroughly combined.

3 Toss the chicken mixture with the dressing and pepper to taste until well combined. Chill in the refrigerator for 1 hour.

4 Divide the chicken salad among the lettuce leaves, roll up, and serve immediately.

PER SERVING: 274 calories (93 from fat), 35 g protein, 10 g fat (2 g saturated fat), 11 g carbohydrates, 2 g fiber, 104 mg cholesterol, 821 mg sodium

Barbecue Chicken Wraps

Think Wild, Wild West for these wraps and use Mountain Bread corn wraps if you can find them in your market. If not, whole wheat tortillas will certainly do the trick. I make my own Barbecue Sauce (opposite page), but if you are going to use store-bought, look for Bull's-Eye brand: It doesn't contain high fructose corn syrup.

4 boneless, skinless chicken breast halves (6 ounces each), cooked and cut into $1/2$-inch cubes

2 celery stalks, chopped

1 cup frozen corn kernels, thawed

$1/2$ cup chopped cilantro

3 tablespoons diced red onion

$1/2$ cup homemade Barbecue Sauce (recipe follows) or store-bought

2 tablespoons fat-free mayonnaise

4 Mountain Bread corn wraps or whole wheat tortillas (8-inch), warmed

Sliced tomatoes and lettuce (optional)

1 Mix the chicken, celery, corn, cilantro, and red onion together in a large bowl. Set aside.

2 Mix the barbecue sauce and mayonnaise together in a small bowl until thoroughly combined.

3 Toss the chicken mixture with the barbecue-mayo sauce until well combined and chill in the refrigerator for 1 hour.

4 Arrange one-quarter of the chicken mixture in the center of each tortilla, leaving a $1/2$-inch border on the sides and bottom. Add lettuce and tomato, if using. Fold the bottom end of the tortilla up and over the filling, fold in both sides, and continue rolling.

PER SERVING: 427 calories (58 from fat), 42 g protein, 6 g fat (1 g saturated fat), 51 g carbohydrates, 5 g fiber, 110 mg cholesterol, 988 mg sodium

BARBECUE SAUCE

MAKES ABOUT 2 CUPS

1 cup natural ketchup, such as Muir Glen

2 tablespoons apple cider vinegar

2 teaspoons fresh lemon juice

2 teaspoons honey

1 teaspoon tomato paste

1 teaspoon Worcestershire sauce

1 teaspoon liquid smoke

1 tablespoon onion powder

1 tablespoon garlic powder

$1/4$ teaspoon freshly ground black pepper

$1/8$ teaspoon ground allspice

$1/8$ teaspoon mustard powder

1 Combine all the ingredients in a saucepan. Bring to a simmer over medium-high heat. Reduce the heat and cook for 5 minutes, whisking occasionally to make a smooth sauce.

2 Let cool. Pour into a glass jar or plastic container and refrigerate for up to 2 weeks.

PER SERVING ($1/4$ cup): 55 calories (0 from fat), 0 g protein, 0 g fat (0 g saturated fat), 12 g carbohydrates, 0.5 g fiber, 0 mg cholesterol, 469 mg sodium

Ready! Action! Energy!

Training stars and getting them into shape for action movies is fun and challenging. I've prepared Jessica Biel, Jennifer Lopez, Winona Ryder, and Jennifer Love Hewitt for super tough action roles. What does it take? A lot of endurance training, strength and power training, plyometrics, cardiovascular training, and, in some cases, water training. And, of course, eating the right foods.

Action scenes require overall body strength and flexibility. Love curled 20-pound dumbbells while training for *The Tuxedo* with Jackie Chan. During certain scenes, she was strapped into a harness to make it look as if she were flying. She was bruised all over from the cables, but she's one tough woman. I amped up her nutrition plan with complex carbs and fruit in the morning and lean proteins throughout the day. I whipped up soy protein shakes for her several times a day, to give her added protein and complex carbs to endure the long days. She kept up her trademark smile the whole time.

Chinese Chicken Salad Rolls

★ :: **MAKES 4**

Most Chinese chicken salads are drenched with sugary dressing and canned mandarin oranges. Not mine! This Asian delight is filled with fresh fruits and veggies, and the tangy dressing is sweetened with Truvia, a natural sweetener made from the stevia plant. You can find Truvia in grocery stores everywhere.

1/3 cup rice vinegar

1/4 cup low-sodium soy sauce

2 tablespoons fresh orange juice

2 teaspoons toasted sesame oil

1 1/2 teaspoons chile sauce, such as Sriracha

1 1/2 teaspoons Truvia

1 teaspoon minced garlic

1 teaspoon minced fresh ginger

4 boneless, skinless chicken breast halves (6 ounces each), cooked and shredded

1 1/2 cups shredded napa cabbage

1 1/2 cups shredded red cabbage

3 scallions, minced

1 can (8 ounces) water chestnuts, rinsed, drained, and chopped

1/4 cup sliced almonds, toasted

1 navel orange, divided into segments

1/4 cup chopped cilantro

4 whole wheat tortillas (8-inch), warmed

1 Whisk together the vinegar, soy sauce, orange juice, sesame oil, chile sauce, Truvia, garlic, and ginger in a bowl. Set aside.

2 Mix together the chicken, cabbages, scallions, water chestnuts, almonds, orange segments, and cilantro in a large bowl. Toss well. Whisk the vinaigrette again and toss with the chicken salad.

3 Spread one-quarter of the chicken salad in the middle of each tortilla, leaving a 1/2-inch border on the sides and bottom. Fold the bottom end of the tortilla up and over the filling, fold in both sides, and continue rolling. Serve.

PER SERVING: 449 calories (103 from fat), 44 g protein, 12 g fat (2 g saturated fat), 43 g carbohydrates, 8 g fiber, 109 mg cholesterol, 1,097 mg sodium

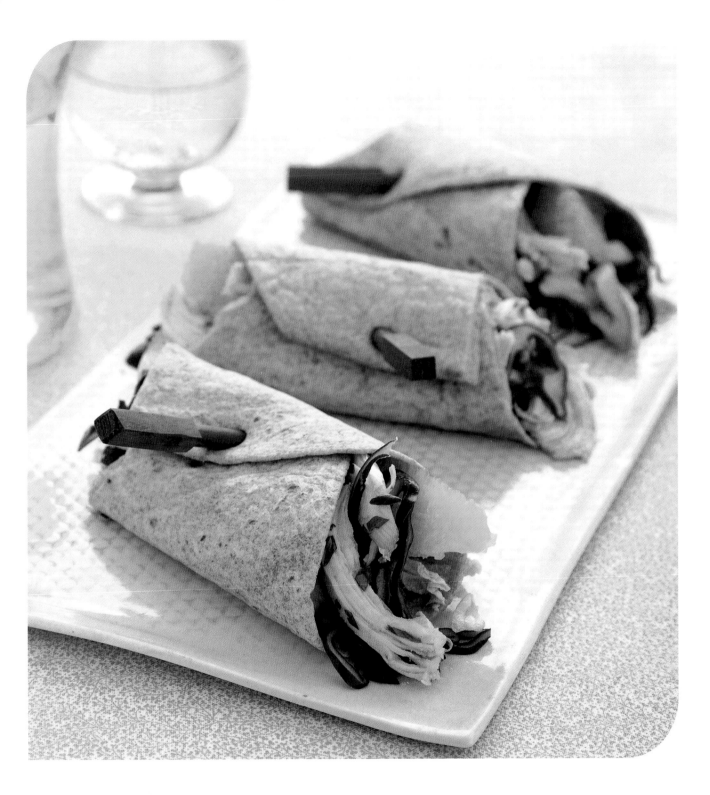

Chicken Tzatziki Wraps

Tzatziki is a garlicky Greek cucumber-yogurt sauce traditionally used as a dip with vegetables or drizzled on grilled fish. I find it fabulously fitting on this chicken wrap. Stir it up with nonfat plain Greek yogurt, which is thick and has just the right tart flavor.

½ cup 0% plain Greek yogurt

½ cucumber, peeled and diced

3 garlic cloves, minced

2 teaspoons extra-virgin olive oil

½ medium onion, diced

4 boneless, skinless chicken breast halves (6 ounces each), cooked and diced

1 teaspoon lemon-pepper

½ teaspoon dried oregano

¼ teaspoon ground allspice

4 whole wheat pocketless pitas (8-inch)

1 Mix together the yogurt, cucumber, and one-third of the minced garlic in a bowl. Cover and refrigerate the tzatziki for 1 hour. It can be made a day ahead.

2 Heat the oil in a skillet over medium heat. Add the onion and the remaining garlic and cook until the onion is softened, 3 to 4 minutes. Add the chicken, lemon-pepper, oregano, and allspice and stir to heat through.

3 Divide the chicken among the 4 pitas, top with the tzatziki, and serve.

PER SERVING: 382 calories (74 from fat), 45 g protein, 8 g fat (1 g saturated fat), 31 g carbohydrates, 5 g fiber, 109 mg cholesterol, 599 mg sodium

Chicken-Cashew Salad Wraps

To preserve the crunch of this nutty chicken salad, stir in the cashews at the last minute so they don't marinate too much in the dressing. To serve as a main course, omit the lavash and spoon the chicken-cashew mixture on some brown rice instead. Add some fruity sweetness with a side of mango-peach salsa.

¼ cup fat-free mayonnaise

1 tablespoon fat-free sour cream

¼ teaspoon curry powder

4 boneless, skinless chicken breast halves (6 ounces each), cooked and diced

⅓ cup chopped celery

¼ cup alfalfa sprouts

2 tablespoons chopped dry-roasted cashews

1 tablespoon chopped scallions

4 pieces (8 x 8-inch) whole wheat lavash

1 Whisk together the mayonnaise, sour cream, and curry powder in a large bowl. Add the chicken, celery, sprouts, cashews, and scallions. Mix well.

2 Divide the chicken salad among the lavash squares. Roll up, folding in the sides, and serve.

PER SERVING: 345 calories (80 from fat), 41 g protein, 9 g fat (1.5 g saturated fat), 27 g carbohydrates, 5 g fiber, 111 mg cholesterol, 361 mg sodium

You Need a Cooler Bag

I'm not talking Prada. I'm talking about a small insulated cooler bag that goes with you to work, school, the playground, etc. We can't live on wraps alone, can we? Take a mini-cooler packed with your own goodies from home to keep you from eating foods that you shouldn't when cravings and hunger set in. Pack your wraps, nonfat yogurt, roasted unsalted almonds, edamame, a banana, hard-boiled egg whites, and an apple.

Cobb Salad Wraps

I make my skinny version of the traditional Cobb salad with turkey bacon, egg whites, and goat cheese—all of which pack more health benefits than the classic ingredients. Watch out, this colorful concoction might just become one of your favorite salads to roll into a wrap!

4 turkey bacon strips

½ cup extra-virgin olive oil

4 teaspoons fresh lemon juice

4 teaspoons Dijon mustard

2 teaspoons red wine vinegar

2 teaspoons balsamic vinegar

2 hard-boiled eggs, peeled

6 cups chopped romaine lettuce + 4 large leaves, center ribs cut out

4 boneless, skinless chicken breast halves (6 ounces each), cooked and diced

1 Hass avocado, chopped

2 plum tomatoes, chopped

⅓ cup crumbled fresh goat cheese

1 Cook the turkey bacon in a nonstick skillet over medium heat until crisp. Remove the bacon to paper towels to drain. When cool, chop and set aside.

2 Whisk together the oil, lemon juice, mustard, and vinegars in a bowl until blended.

3 Halve the hard-boiled eggs and discard the yolks. Chop the whites into small pieces.

4 Combine the chopped romaine, bacon, egg whites, chicken, avocado, tomatoes, and goat cheese in a bowl and toss well to combine. Whisk the dressing again and toss with the salad ingredients.

5 Spoon the salad onto the romaine leaves, roll up, and serve.

PER SERVING: 634 calories (402 from fat), 50 g protein, 45 g fat (8 g saturated fat), 9 g carbohydrates, 5 g fiber, 245 mg cholesterol, 350 mg sodium

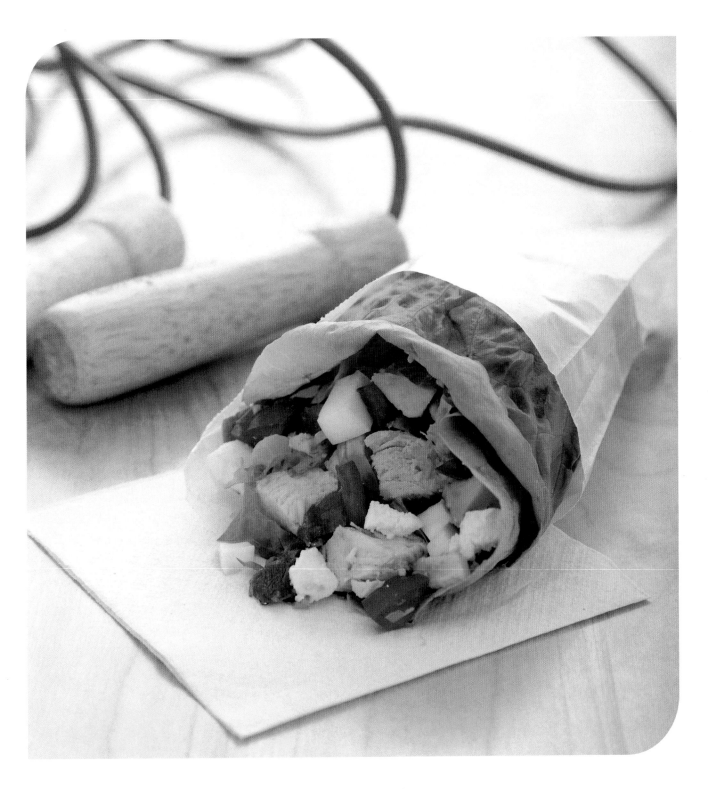

Chicken Wraps *with* Dill Cream Cheese

★ :: **MAKES 4**

These lettuce wraps remind me of the dainty chicken-and-cream-cheese sandwiches served at elegant tea parties. Enjoy them for lunch or at a tea party of your own. The filling can also be spread on wraps or low-carb crackers.

6 ounces fat-free cream cheese, at room temperature

1 tablespoon chopped fresh dill

1 tablespoon minced garlic

4 large butter lettuce leaves

4 boneless, skinless chicken breast halves (6 ounces each), cooked and diced

2 small tomatoes, diced

1 Whisk together the cream cheese, dill, and garlic in a bowl.

2 Spread the cream cheese mixture on the lettuce leaves and top with the chicken and tomatoes. Roll up, tucking in the ends, and serve.

PER SERVING: 253 calories (41 from fat), 43 g protein, 5 g fat (1 g saturated fat), 6 g carbohydrates, 1 g fiber, 115 mg cholesterol, 505 mg sodium

STAY HOLLYWOOD SLIM WHEN EATING OUT

★ ★ ★ ★ ★ ★ ★ ★ ★ ★ ★ ★ ★ ★ ★ ★ ★

Eating out should be about relaxing, socializing, and trying fun, new foods, but take care not to sabotage all your hard work once you sit down and open up that menu. I've accompanied many a celeb to restaurants while on location and have taught them how to negotiate a menu and eat a satisfying meal that won't undermine their star appeal when they get in front of the camera. Menu descriptions can be misleading: Broiled chicken and grilled fish sound healthy, but they're not if topped with cheese or a creamy sauce. Don't be shy about asking for what you want—you're paying for it.

When you're hungry and walk into a restaurant, it's so tempting to dive into that basket of bread and butter, so have the bread basket removed immediately. I don't even let the waiter put it on the table. The same goes for tortilla chips. If you are really ravenous and can't wait for your entree, ask for some warm corn tortillas instead. Dipping these into fresh salsa is just as satisfying as loading up on the fried kind.

As soon as you sit down, order a mixed salad with dressing on the side, or a broth-based soup, or fresh fruit or vegetables, or a light, fresh seafood appetizer like shrimp or crab cocktail. These will take the edge off your hunger right away. Use salad dressings sparingly, or ask for olive oil and lemon wedges and/or balsamic vinegar. Dressings made with low-fat buttermilk are another good alternative, but avoid ranch and blue cheese dressings—they're loaded with fat.

Order your protein dish—chicken, meat, or best of all, fish—grilled, steamed, baked, or broiled without sauce and avoid anything sautéed or fried. The same goes for vegetables: Ask for them steamed or grilled with lemon juice, Dijon mustard, olive oil, and vinegar as condiments. Trim excess fat from red meat and remove the skin from poultry. Watch your portions. Restaurant portions are just huge these days! As soon as my main course arrives, I set aside half to take home for another meal. You could also order 2 apps or just share a main course with a friend.

Drink still or sparkling water with your meal rather than soda or wine. In fact, avoid alcohol as much as possible, especially creamy drinks, sweet cocktails, and fruity drinks like margaritas. If you must indulge, limit yourself to one glass of red or white wine and alternate sips of wine and water.

Lastly, never stuff yourself. When you expand your tummy, you expand your appetite.

Chicken-Asparagus Wraps

★ :: **MAKES 4**

When I trained Steven Spielberg, he absolutely loved this flavorful chicken and asparagus salad. So, I thought, why not put it in a wrap? Make sure to use fresh curry powder to achieve the proper level of spice. If it's been in your cabinet for more than 6 months, buy a new container.

2 tablespoons sliced almonds

½ pound asparagus

½ cup fat-free mayonnaise

2 teaspoons curry powder

1 teaspoon fresh lemon juice

Freshly ground black pepper

4 boneless, skinless chicken breast halves (6 ounces each), cooked and diced

⅔ cup chopped red bell pepper

¼ cup chopped parsley

4 pieces (8 x 8-inch) whole wheat lavash

1. Place the almonds in a skillet over medium-high heat. Shake the nuts continuously until they start to turn color, 3 to 5 minutes. Remove immediately from the heat and set aside.

2. Fill a bowl with ice and water. Bring ½ inch water to a boil in a skillet. Add the asparagus, cover, reduce the heat, and simmer until the asparagus are cooked but still firm, 1½ to 2 minutes. Using tongs, remove the asparagus to the bowl of ice water to stop the cooking. Drain and dry the asparagus and cut into 1-inch pieces.

3. Whisk together the mayonnaise, curry powder, lemon juice, and black pepper to taste in a large bowl.

4. Add the asparagus, almonds, chicken, bell pepper, and parsley, tossing well to coat with the dressing.

5. Divide the chicken-asparagus mixture among the lavash squares. Roll up, tucking in both ends on the sides, and serve.

PER SERVING: 364 calories (81 from fat), 42 g protein, 9 g fat (1 g saturated fat), 32 g carbohydrates, 7 g fiber, 112 mg cholesterol, 471 mg sodium

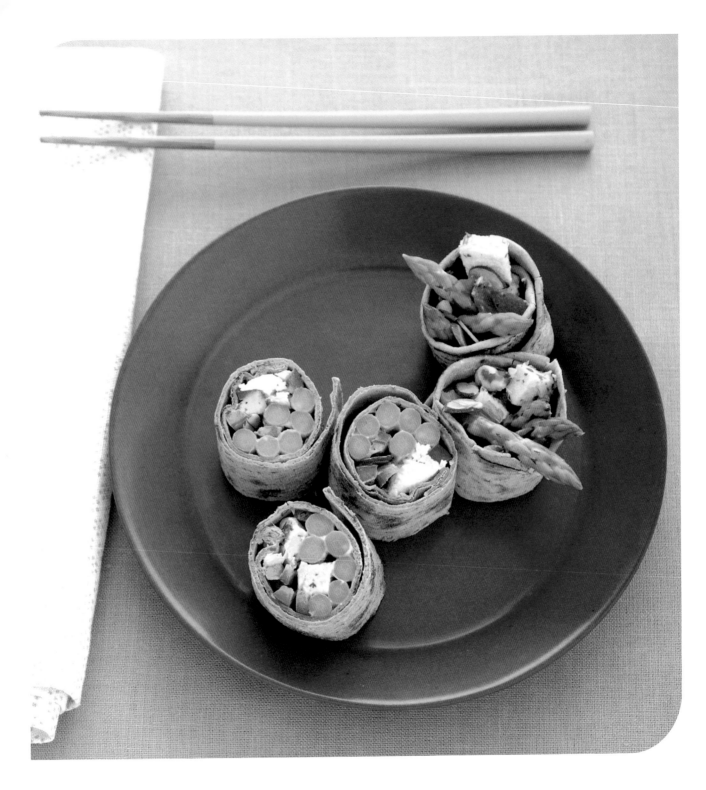

Chicken Caesar Wraps

Caesar salads are an American restaurant favorite . . . and usually a minefield of fat and calories. Skip the table service and enjoy your Caesar with the chicken, low-fat dressing, and shredded romaine lettuce in this virtuous Hollywood package.

2 tablespoons fat-free mayonnaise

2 tablespoons grated Parmesan cheese

1/2 teaspoon anchovy paste

1 garlic clove, chopped

1 teaspoon Dijon mustard

1 1/2 teaspoons fresh lemon juice

4 whole wheat tortillas (8-inch)

4 boneless, skinless chicken breast halves (6 ounces each), cooked and sliced

1/2 head romaine lettuce, shredded

1 Whisk together the mayonnaise, Parmesan, anchovy paste, garlic, mustard, and lemon juice in a bowl.

2 Spread each tortilla with the dressing and top with the chicken and lettuce. Fold the bottom end of the tortilla up and over the filling, fold in both sides, and continue rolling. Serve.

PER SERVING: 364 calories (70 from fat), 42 g protein, 8 g fat (2 g saturated fat), 30 g carbohydrates, 5 g fiber, 115 mg cholesterol, 684 mg sodium

Indonesian Chicken Wraps

The sesame chicken for these exotic lettuce wraps gets a double dip of peanutty batter and a sesame crust that is oh so delicious. Think about using rice papers as wrappers, too. Serve with Asian-inspired coleslaw of Chinese cabbage, shredded carrots, scallions, cilantro, and a light dressing.

2 tablespoons low-sodium soy sauce

1 tablespoon smooth unsalted peanut butter

2 teaspoons toasted sesame oil

Juice of ½ lime

¼ cup unbleached all-purpose flour

3 tablespoons sesame seeds

⅛ teaspoon freshly ground black pepper

4 boneless, skinless chicken breast halves (6 ounces each)

8 romaine lettuce leaves, center ribs cut out

1 Preheat the oven to 450°F. Coat a baking dish large enough to hold the chicken in a single layer with cooking spray.

2 Combine the soy sauce, peanut butter, sesame oil, and lime juice in a blender or food processor. Blend until smooth. Pour onto a plate. On another plate, mix together the flour, sesame seeds, and pepper.

3 Dip a chicken breast in the peanut butter mixture to coat. Then dip it into the flour mixture, shaking off the excess. Put the chicken in the baking dish. Repeat with the other chicken breasts.

4 Bake the chicken for 20 to 25 minutes, or until cooked through.

5 When cool enough to handle, slice the chicken breasts, place on top of the lettuce leaves, and serve warm, 2 per person.

PER SERVING: 312 calories (16 from fat), 40 g protein, 12 g fat (2 g saturated fat), 9 g carbohydrates, 1 g fiber, 109 mg cholesterol, 479 mg sodium

Chicken *and* Salsa Wraps

★ :: MAKES 4

Boneless, skinless chicken breasts are the go-to for a lot of girls watching their figures. But plain chicken is SO boring! Homemade salsa totally perks up the poultry in this super healthy wrap. And no need to be stingy with the salsa—it's low in calories and has no fat!

½ cup Salsa Picante (page 39)

¼ cup Dijon mustard

¼ cup fresh lime juice + 4 lime wedges

1 teaspoon dried dillweed

4 boneless, skinless chicken breast halves (6 ounces each)

1 tablespoon extra-virgin olive oil

¼ cup fat-free sour cream

4 whole wheat tortillas (8-inch), warmed

1 Mix together the salsa, mustard, lime juice, and dillweed in a bowl. Remove ¾ cup salsa and set aside. Add the chicken to the bowl with the remaining salsa mixture. Toss well. Cover the bowl with plastic wrap and refrigerate for 30 minutes.

2 Heat the oil in a large skillet over medium heat. Remove the chicken from the salsa marinade and discard the marinade. Add the chicken to the hot skillet and cook on each side for 5 minutes. Add the reserved ¾ cup salsa to the skillet, cover, and cook until the chicken is cooked through, another 8 minutes. Remove the chicken to a plate and let sit for 5 minutes so its juices can be reabsorbed, then slice thinly.

3 Spread 1 tablespoon of sour cream on each tortilla and top with some sliced chicken breast. Roll and serve with a wedge of lime.

PER SERVING: 393 calories (87 from fat), 41 g protein, 10 g fat (2 g saturated fat), 35 g carbohydrates, 4 g fiber, 110 mg cholesterol, 686 mg sodium

Orange-Ginger Chicken Wraps

★ :: **MAKES 4**

Anyone for a helping of healthy Chinese food? While the orange chicken from the local take-out place is deep-fried and oily, my recipe uses fresh oranges and ginger and is thickened with a little bit of arrowroot. Fabulous flavor without fat and freaky additives? Yes please!

1½ cups orange juice

1½ tablespoons arrowroot

2 teaspoons extra-virgin olive oil

1 red bell pepper, cored, seeded, and chopped

1 pound boneless, skinless chicken breasts, cut into ½-inch pieces

1 navel orange, divided into segments

½ cup chopped scallions

3 tablespoons hoisin sauce

2 teaspoons grated orange zest

1 teaspoon minced fresh ginger

1 garlic clove, minced

⅛ teaspoon crushed red pepper flakes

1 teaspoon rice vinegar

¼ cup cashews, chopped

4 whole wheat tortillas (8-inch), warmed

1 In a small bowl, combine 3 tablespoons of the orange juice and the arrowroot and whisk together until dissolved.

2 Heat the oil in a large skillet over medium-high heat. Add the bell pepper and chicken and stir-fry until the chicken is no longer pink, 5 to 6 minutes.

3 Add the orange segments, scallions, hoisin sauce, orange zest, ginger, garlic, red pepper flakes, rice vinegar, arrowroot mixture, and the remaining orange juice and and mix well. Bring to a boil, then reduce the heat to a simmer and cook until the sauce thickens, 5 to 6 minutes.

4 Add the cashews. Divide evenly among the tortillas, roll, and serve.

PER SERVING: 461 calories (102 from fat), 31 g protein, 11 g fat (2 g saturated fat), 59 g carbohydrates, 6 g fiber, 73 mg cholesterol, 783 mg sodium

Tandoori Chicken Wraps

Boy oh boy, did Kevin Costner love this Indian-inspired wrap. The chicken is marinated in yogurt and spices before being cooked, so no additional sauce is necessary. Serve with a vinegary cucumber salad and finish it off with some sliced papaya for a fresh, jungle twist.

1 cup 0% plain Greek yogurt

1 teaspoon ground coriander

1 teaspoon turmeric

½ teaspoon paprika

¼ teaspoon ground cardamom

¼ teaspoon ground cumin

Grated zest of 1 lime

1½ pounds boneless, skinless chicken breasts, cut into 1-inch pieces

½ cup frozen peas and carrots, thawed

4 whole wheat naan

1 Whisk together the yogurt, coriander, turmeric, paprika, cardamom, cumin, and lime zest in a shallow baking dish. Add the chicken, stir to coat, cover, and marinate for 20 to 30 minutes in the refrigerator.

2 Heat a skillet over high heat. Coat with cooking spray. Put the chicken and marinade in the skillet and cook until the chicken is cooked through, 6 to 7 minutes. Add the peas and carrots and cook for 2 or 3 minutes to heat through.

3 Spoon the chicken and sauce onto the naan, roll around the filling, and serve.

PER SERVING: 537 calories (104 from fat), 52 g protein, 12 g fat (3 g saturated fat), 61 g carbohydrates, 7 g fiber, 119 mg cholesterol, 233 mg sodium

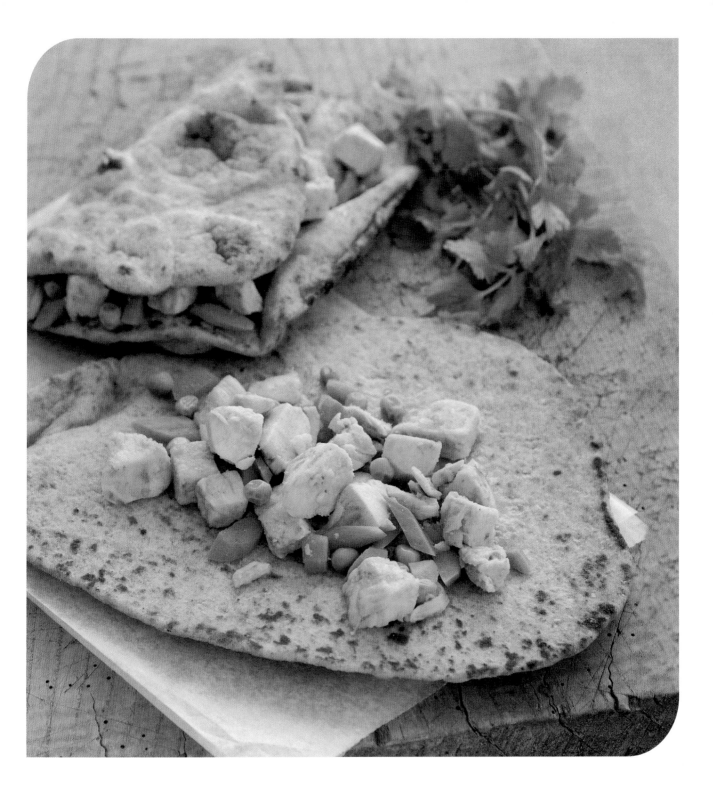

Grilled Chicken Wraps *with* Honey-Mustard-Dill Sauce

You can't go wrong pairing chicken with mushrooms. To make these wraps even more filling and nutritious, add ¼ cup of cooked brown rice to each. Some steamed asparagus on the side adds a splash of color and crunch.

2 tablespoons Dijon mustard

2 tablespoons chopped fresh dill

1 teaspoon honey

¾ cup nonfat plain yogurt

Freshly ground black pepper

4 boneless, skinless chicken breast halves (6 ounces each)

1 teaspoon olive oil

8 ounces white mushrooms, sliced

2 plum tomatoes, chopped

4 honey-wheat tortillas (8-inch)

1 Whisk together the mustard, dill, honey, yogurt, and pepper in a bowl. Set aside.

2 Coat a skillet with cooking spray and place over high heat. Add the chicken and cook until cooked through, 5 to 7 minutes on each side. Using tongs, remove the chicken to a plate. Let the chicken rest for 5 to 8 minutes until the juices are reabsorbed, then thinly slice across the grain.

3 Heat the oil in the same skillet. Add the mushrooms and cook, stirring occasionally, until tender, 5 to 7 minutes. Add the honey-mustard-dill sauce and tomatoes and simmer for 5 minutes.

4 Divide the chicken slices among the tortillas. Top with the mushrooms and sauce. Fold the bottom end of the tortilla up and over the filling, fold in both sides, and continue rolling. Serve.

PER SERVING: 358 calories (69 from fat), 42 g protein, 8 g fat (1 g saturated fat), 32 g carbohydrates, 2 g fiber, 110 mg cholesterol, 423 mg sodium

Two Weeks to a Bikini Body

What to do about that muffin top around your waist when your sun-and-fun vacation is just two weeks away?

Here's what I tell my stars and other celeb clients: Work out. A lot. Sweat. A lot. And then work out some more. Saddle up on the cardio cycle or walk the treadmill twice a day for a minimum of 45 minutes. Burn fat by kicking up your weight-lifting routine and trying something new like jogging instead of riding the stationary bike. Then try these tips.

★ Drink nothing but water or green tea. No soda, no coffee, no juice, no alcohol. I mean it.

★ Reduce the number of calories you consume by 10 to 20 percent.

★ Watch portion size carefully.

★ Do not skip breakfast; it's the most important meal of the day.

★ Take a good multivitamin daily.

★ Get a little bit of sun.

★ Eat lots of asparagus. It's a natural diuretic.

★ Skip all white foods. For the next two weeks, sugar, flour, pasta, and breads don't exist as far as you're concerned.

★ Eat lots of vegetables, salads, and fruit. Eat lightly but often. I make sure my clients eat four to five small meals throughout the day. Have a soy protein drink or a sliced apple with a little nut butter in midafternoon to boost your energy levels.

With this super-mini-going-on-vacation-boot-camp, your belly—and the rest of you—will be flatter and tighter. Instead of hiding your bod under an XXL T-shirt, you'll strut down the beach without a cover-up. But with a smile and attitude.

Chicken *with* Broccoli *and* Snow Peas Wraps

★ :: **MAKES 4**

Another Chinese restaurant favorite made healthy and rolled up into a wrap! Keep bags—not boxes—of frozen broccoli, snow peas, and other vegetables on hand, so you can dip in and take out just what you need. This chicken with veggies can also be served atop a scoop of steamed brown rice.

½ **cup frozen broccoli florets**

½ **cup frozen snow peas**

¾ **cup canned chickpeas, rinsed and drained**

1 **can (8 ounces) water chestnuts, rinsed, drained, and chopped**

2 **tablespoons seasoned rice vinegar**

2 **tablespoons low-sodium soy sauce**

1½ **tablespoons olive oil**

1 **tablespoon honey**

2 **tablespoons sesame seeds**

1 **cup diced cooked boneless, skinless chicken breast**

4 **spinach-flavored whole wheat tortillas (8-inch), warmed**

1 Cook the broccoli and snow peas as directed on the packages. Drain and set aside.

2 Combine the chickpeas, water chestnuts, vinegar, soy sauce, oil, honey, and sesame seeds in a saucepan. Bring to a simmer over medium heat. Stir in the chicken and vegetables and cook until heated through and any liquid is absorbed. Set aside to cool slightly.

3 Spread one-quarter of the chicken mixture in the middle of each tortilla, leaving a ½-inch border on the sides and bottom. Fold the bottom end of the tortilla up and over the filling, fold in both sides, and continue rolling. Serve.

PER SERVING: 570 calories (180 from fat), 24 g protein, 21 g fat (3 g saturated fat), 73 g carbohydrates, 8 g fiber, 30 mg cholesterol, 1,020 mg sodium

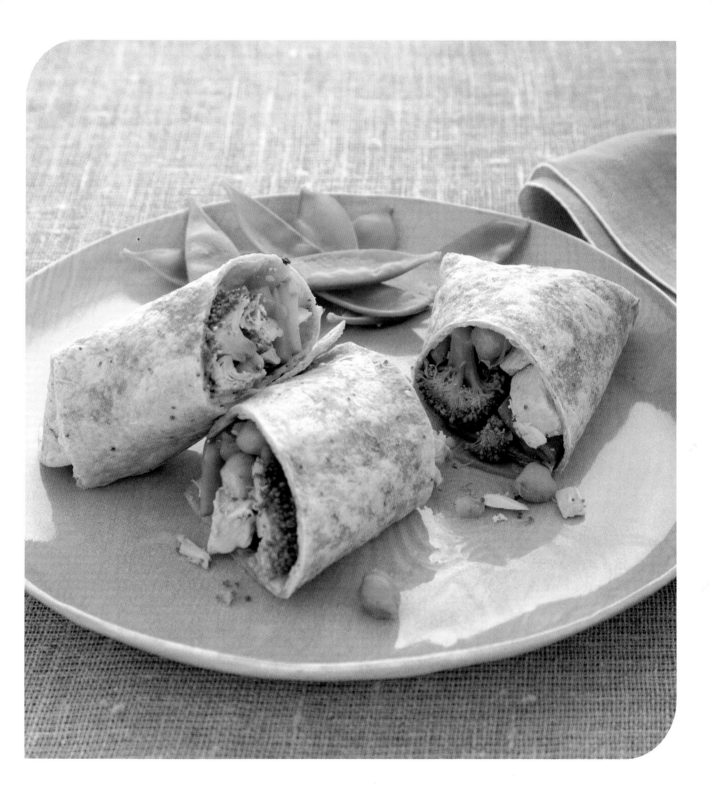

Chicken Fajitas Wraps

Chicken fajitas are a Hollywood favorite. I prepare them for my clients with a little bit of chipotle peppers in adobo sauce (smoked jalapeños in a red sauce). Look for this spicy condiment in the Latin food section of your supermarket. If you have some leftover, put two chipotles plus a little bit of the adobo sauce into each compartment of an ice-cube tray and freeze. Then, store the cubes in a resealable plastic bag in the freezer, and you'll have Mexican sauces at the ready for up to 2 months!

4 boneless, skinless chicken breast halves (6 ounces each), cooked and cut into strips

2 chipotles in adobo sauce, minced

1 tablespoon extra-virgin olive oil

2 garlic cloves, minced

2 red bell peppers, cut into strips

1 small red onion, sliced

2 tablespoons fat-free sour cream

4 whole wheat tortillas (8-inch)

Dried oregano

1 Mix the chicken and chipotles together in a bowl. Set aside.

2 Heat the oil in a skillet over medium heat. Add the garlic, peppers, and onion and cook until the vegetables are soft, 8 to 10 minutes. Add the cooked vegetables to the chicken and toss to combine.

3 Smear ½ tablespoon sour cream on each tortilla, then top with the chicken and a pinch of dried oregano. Fold the bottom end of the tortilla up and over the filling, fold in both sides, and continue rolling. Serve warm.

PER SERVING: 395 calories (90 from fat), 41 g protein, 10 g fat (2 g saturated fat), 33 g carbohydrates, 5 g fiber, 110 mg cholesterol, 571 mg sodium

Working Out on the Road

Working out away from home can be a real challenge. It's just as difficult for my clients to find the time and a good facility for working out on the road as it is for you.

Finding time to exercise in your busy schedule when meetings and appointments start early and run late isn't easy. At the end of a long, stressful day, about all you want to do is order room service and a movie! You don't have to do a full workout every day, but make an effort to do *something* to maintain your fitness level. Here are some tips for working out on the road.

1. Select a hotel with an on-site gym. Ask how much equipment is in the gym and what type it is. It's depressing to roll out of bed with good workout intentions only to find that the "gym" is a closet with a broken-down bike and 3-pound weights.

2. Some hotels have deals with gyms that are nearby and within walking distance. I like to visit gyms when I travel to see what others are doing, and there's always great people-watching.

3. If you're a runner, ask the concierge or desk clerk for a running map. Stay on the recommended route.

4. Some luxury hotels will provide a bike, treadmill, or elliptical trainer in your room for a nominal charge. If your room doesn't have a mini-fridge, request one so you can have bottled water, yogurt, fruit, and other healthy snacks on hand. If you can't stand the temptation, have the minibar removed.

5. Pack some resistance bands. They take up very little room in your suitcase.

Following are a few easy workout moves you can do anytime, anywhere—no gym required!

★ March in place for 3 to 5 minutes to elevate your heart rate.

★ Clasp your hands and extend them out in front of your chest to stretch your back. Hold for 5 seconds.

★ Clasp your hands behind your back, extending them backward, opening up your chest.

★ Cross one foot in front of the other, while softening your knees. Raise your hands above your head and take a deep breath. Slowly lower your arms and head toward the ground as you exhale. Try to touch the floor, taking care not to bounce. Hold for 15 seconds, rise to standing and switch feet. Bend and stretch as before.

★ Lie on the floor with your knees bent and your feet flat on the floor. Slowly lift your pelvis up and squeeze your booty. Keep your abs tight and hold for one count. Slowly lower yourself to the start position. Repeat 25 times, rest for 30 seconds, and then do another 25. Make this exercise more challenging by raising one leg or by coming up on your heels.

★ Lie on the floor with your knees bent and legs together. Drop your legs to one side. Using both hands to hold a filled water bottle or dumbbell out in front of you, lift your shoulders a few inches off the floor by contracting your abs. Contract and partially release your oblique muscles—the ab muscles that run up the sides of your waist—25 times. Shift your legs to the other side and repeat the exercise.

Chicken Parm Wraps

This is my lightened version of classic Italian-American chicken Parmigiana. The traditional recipe includes chicken cutlets that are breaded and fried, then baked covered in tomato sauce and a layer of cheese. And it's usually served with a side of spaghetti! Time-consuming to make, and super caloric to eat. These chicken parm Hollywood Wraps are delicious, quick-to-prepare, and nutritionally sound. Consider making them for your next Super Bowl or other sports party.

4 whole wheat tortillas (8-inch), pesto garlic-flavored or plain

4 boneless, skinless chicken breast halves (6 ounces each), cooked and diced

2 plum tomatoes, diced

1 cup roasted red peppers, sliced

4 ounces fat-free mozzarella, cut into 4 slices

4 teaspoons extra-virgin olive oil

½ cup grated Parmesan cheese

8 fresh basil leaves, shredded

1 Preheat the oven to 375°F.

2 Arrange the tortillas on a baking sheet. Top with the chicken, tomatoes, roasted peppers, and mozzarella. Drizzle on 1 teaspoon of oil. Sprinkle on the Parmesan.

3 Bake for 3 to 4 minutes, or until the cheese melts.

4 Remove from the oven and top with the basil. Fold the bottom end of the tortilla up and over the filling, fold in both sides, and continue rolling. Serve.

PER SERVING: 499 calories (141 from fat), 53 g protein, 16 g fat (5 g saturated fat), 32 g carbohydrates, 4 g fiber, 134 mg cholesterol, 1,083 mg sodium

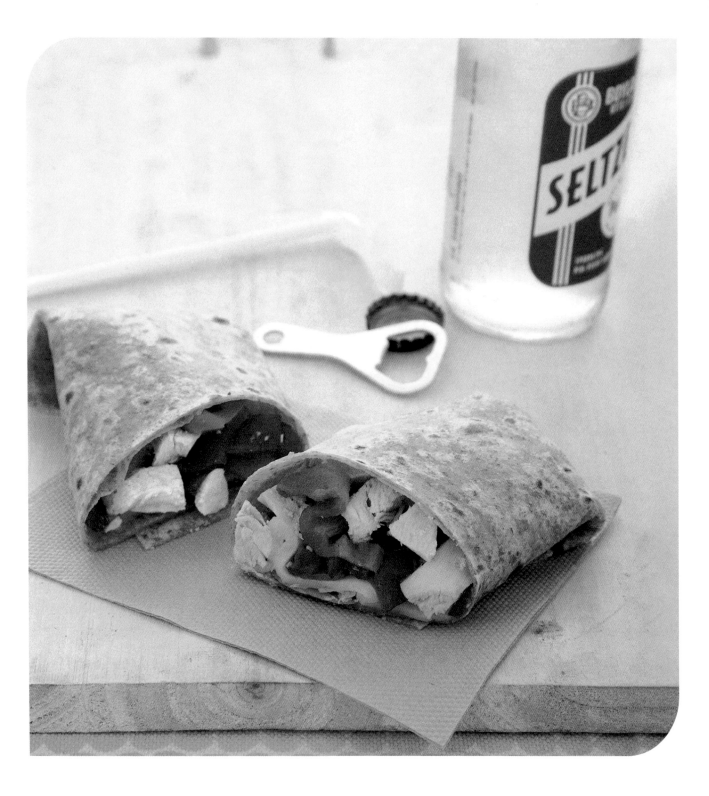

Chicken-Mushroom Wraps *with* Lemon *and* Herbs

★ :: **MAKES 4**

You can go in a lot of cultural directions with these herb-alicious wraps. If there's no lemon juice, oregano, and basil in the kitchen, substitute lime and cilantro for a Mexican-inspired wrap or herbes de Provence for South-of-France flavors.

1 tablespoon extra-virgin olive oil

1 cup sliced white mushrooms

1 tablespoon minced garlic

¼ cup dry white wine

2 tablespoons fresh lemon juice

4 boneless, skinless chicken breast halves (6 ounces each), cooked and diced

¾ cup cooked brown rice

4 whole wheat tortillas (8-inch), warmed

2 plum tomatoes, diced

1 tablespoon chopped fresh basil

1 teaspoon dried oregano

1 Heat the oil in a skillet over medium heat. Add the mushrooms and cook until browned, about 5 minutes.

2 Add the garlic and wine and simmer for 2 to 3 minutes. Add the lemon juice, chicken, and rice. Cook for 5 to 7 minutes, stirring occasionally, to heat through.

3 Divide the chicken and rice mixture among the tortillas and top with the tomatoes, basil, and oregano. Fold the bottom end of the tortilla up and over the filling, fold in both sides, and continue rolling. Serve warm.

PER SERVING: 423 calories (89 from fat), 42 g protein, 10 g fat (1.5 g saturated fat), 38 g carbohydrates, 4 g fiber, 109 mg cholesterol, 533 mg sodium

The Hollywood Wrap

Minced Chicken Lettuce Wraps

Chicken Soong is a classic Chinese dish typically served in lettuce cups (*soong* means "minced" in Mandarin and Cantonese). This version uses far less oil and sodium than one you would get in a take-out container.

1 tablespoon canola oil

1 pound ground chicken breast

1 large onion, finely diced

2 garlic cloves, minced

2 teaspoons minced fresh ginger

1 tablespoon low-sodium soy sauce

1 tablespoon rice vinegar

½ teaspoon Sriracha chili sauce

¼ teaspoon low-sodium soy sauce

1 (8 ounces) water chestnuts, drained, rinsed and finely chopped

1 cup finely sliced scallions

2 teaspoons toasted sesame oil

16 Bibb lettuce leaves

1. Heat the canola oil in a skillet over medium heat. Add the chicken and cook, breaking it up with a spoon, until cooked through and no longer pink, about 12 minutes. Transfer the chicken to a fine-mesh strainer to drain off any oil and liquids, then set aside.

2. In the same skillet, cook the onion over medium heat until soft, 4 to 5 minutes. Add the garlic, ginger, soy sauce, vinegar, chili sauce, and soy sauce. Cook for 2 minutes, stirring frequently until blended.

3. Add the water chestnuts, scallions, and sesame oil and cook until the scallions wilt, about 2 minutes.

4. Return the chicken to the skillet and cook together 10 minutes so the flavors mix in well with the chicken.

5. Divide the chicken mixture among the lettuce leaves and serve 4 per person.

PER SERVING: 269 calories (137 from fat), 22 g protein, 15 g fat (3 g saturated fat), 13 g carbohydrates, 4 g fiber, 98 mg cholesterol, 239 mg sodium

Thanksgiving Turkey Wraps

What to do with all of those Thanksgiving leftovers? That's easy. Use all the goodies—turkey, cranberry sauce, sweet potatoes—to make wraps for lunch the next day.

2 tablespoons cranberry preserves or fresh cranberry sauce

2 tablespoons fat-free mayonnaise

4 honey-wheat tortillas (8 inches)

1 pound roasted turkey breast, thinly sliced

1 baked sweet potato, peeled and cut lengthwise into 4 wedges

1 Stir the cranberry preserves and mayonnaise together in a small bowl, mixing well.

2 Spread the mayonnaise on each tortilla, top each with one-quarter of the turkey and a sweet potato wedge.

3 Fold the bottom end of the tortilla up and over the filling, fold in both sides, and continue rolling. Serve.

PER SERVING: 334 calories (11 from fat), 37 g protein, 6 g fat (1 g saturated fat), 34 g carbohydrates, 3 g fiber, 79 mg cholesterol, 287 mg sodium

★

The Hollywood Wrap

She's Got Legs and Knows How to Use Them

So says the ZZ Top song. Lean, bare legs are all over the red carpet. How do stars get those fabulous gams?

Running is the number one way to get your legs in shape fast. Running builds and tones your glutes, quads, hamstrings, and calves. Start slowly. Just get outside and start walking. Walk briskly for 5 to 7 minutes to warm up, and then pick up some speed with a light jog.

Lunges and deadlifts are the two best exercises for achieving toned movie star legs. Make these part of your daily routine:

★ Lunges with a Medicine Ball

Stand with your feet shoulder-width apart. Hold a medicine ball straight out in front. Step forward with your right leg and drop the back knee down until it is 2 inches from the floor. At the same time, raise the ball directly over your head as you lunge forward, Push back through your heel, off your right front leg, and return to the start position. Repeat on the left side. Always make sure that your front knee does not extend beyond your toes; if it does, step out further. Do 2 sets of 12 on each side.

★ Deadlifts with Dumbbells

Stand with your feet a few inches apart. Hold dumbbells at thigh level with your hands shoulder-width apart. With your shoulders pushed back, chest lifted, and knees slightly bent, bend forward at the waist and lower the dumbbells to the floor in a controlled movement. When you feel a good stretch in the back of your legs, stop and hold your position for a moment. Slowly return to a standing position. Squeeze your glutes for 5 seconds. Pay close attention to your form. Don't round your back and be sure to face forward. Don't "use" your back or spine to execute movement. Keep your legs in place but avoid locking your knees.

Always keep your abs tight when doing any exercise to protect your lower back, and don't forget to breathe!

Pumpkin-Turkey Chili Wraps

★ :: MAKES 4

Canned pumpkin puree adds a burst of flavor and health benefits to this hearty autumn dish. This chili can be made ahead, refrigerated, and then reheated, or packed into 1-cup containers and frozen.

1 teaspoon olive oil

1 pound extra-lean ground turkey breast

$\frac{1}{2}$ cup diced onion

$\frac{1}{2}$ cup diced red bell pepper

1 can (15 ounces) red kidney beans, rinsed and drained

2 cups no-salt-added tomato juice

1 can (14$\frac{1}{2}$ ounces) no-salt-added diced tomatoes

1$\frac{1}{4}$ cups (10 ounces) canned unsweetened pumpkin puree

1 tablespoon maple syrup

1$\frac{1}{2}$ teaspoons pumpkin pie spice

1$\frac{1}{2}$ teaspoons chili powder

$\frac{1}{4}$ teaspoon grated nutmeg

$\frac{1}{4}$ cup fat-free sour cream

4 honey-wheat tortillas (8-inch), warmed

1 Heat the oil in a large nonstick skillet. Add the turkey and cook, stirring frequently, until the meat loses its raw color.

2 Stir in the onion and bell pepper and cook until softened, about 5 minutes. Stir in the beans, tomato juice, diced tomatoes, pumpkin, and maple syrup. Add the pumpkin pie spice, chili powder, and nutmeg and mix well. Bring to a boil, reduce to a simmer, and cook, uncovered, for 45 minutes, or until most of the juices are absorbed.

3 Divide the mixture among the tortillas and add 1 tablespoon of sour cream. Fold the bottom end of the tortilla up and over the filling, fold in both sides, and continue rolling. Serve.

PER SERVING: 431 calories (53 from fat), 40 g protein, 6 g fat (0.5 g saturated fat), 60 g carbohydrates, 11 g fiber, 46 mg cholesterol, 404 mg sodium

I became famous for this chili while cooking for Kevin Costner on the set of *For the Love of the Game*. Whenever I made it, other cast and crew members asked, "What's that delicious smell coming from Kevin's trailer?" I was soon making big pots of chili to share with Kelly Preston and the rest of the team.

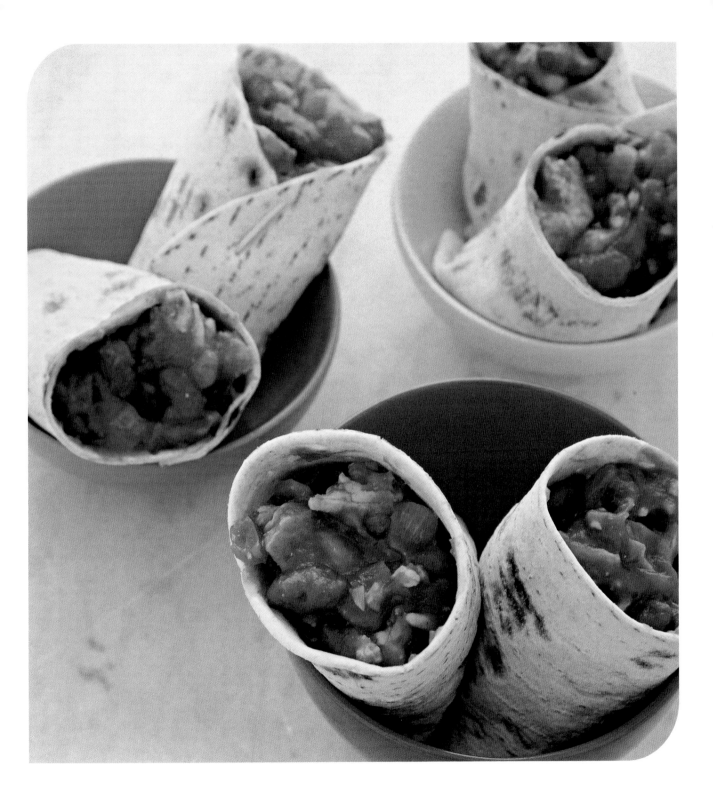

Turkey Quesadillas

Quesadillas are certainly delicious, but they are often made with several tortillas and filled with enough high-fat cheese to undo your entire day. I use just one tortilla, turkey, and low-fat cheeses to lighten them up.

4 whole wheat tortillas (8-inch)

½ cup crumbled fat-free feta

½ cup shredded fat-free Cheddar cheese

1 pound sliced low-sodium turkey breast

¼ cup Salsa Picante (page 39)

1 Hass avocado, sliced

1 Coat a skillet with cooking spray and heat the skillet over medium heat. Put a tortilla in the pan and when just warm, sprinkle with 2 tablespoons each of the feta and Cheddar. When the cheeses are slightly melted, top with one-quarter of the turkey. Cook for about 1 minute. Remove from the pan and top with 1 tablespoon salsa and one-quarter of the avocado. Set aside to cool slightly, then roll up and serve warm.

2 Repeat with the remaining ingredients.

PER SERVING: 326 calories (61 from fat), 34 g protein, 7 g fat (1 g saturated fat), 32 g carbohydrates, 6 g fiber, 55 mg cholesterol, 1,311 mg sodium

Turkey Tacos

Everybody likes his or her taco filled with something a little different. These turkey tacos are basic, but you can accompany them with salsa, shredded fat-free Cheddar, diced tomatoes, avocado, red onions, and your favorite hot sauce. Make sure to purchase ground turkey labeled "extra-lean." Some ground turkey labeled simply "lean" can be just as fattening as ground beef.

1 pound extra-lean ground turkey breast

$1/2$ cup chopped onion

$1^1/4$ cups diced tomatoes

$1/4$ cup canned diced mild green chiles

1 teaspoon chili powder

1 teaspoon ground cumin

$1/2$ teaspoon dried oregano

4 whole wheat tortillas (8-inch), warmed

$1/4$ cup fat-free sour cream

1 Cook the turkey and onion in a large non-stick skillet over medium-high heat, stirring every so often, until the turkey is cooked through and no longer pink, 7 to 10 minutes.

2 Add the tomatoes, chiles, chili powder, cumin, and oregano. Reduce the heat to medium and cook until most of the liquid has evaporated, 3 to 6 minutes.

3 Spread one-quarter of the turkey mixture in the middle of each tortilla, leaving a $1/2$-inch border on the sides and bottom. Top with 1 tablespoon sour cream. Fold the bottom end of the tortilla up and over the filling, fold in both sides, and continue rolling. Serve warm.

PER SERVING: 288 calories (31 from fat), 34 g protein, 3 g fat (0 g saturated fat), 33 g carbohydrates, 5 g fiber, 46 mg cholesterol, 446 mg sodium

BLT Wraps *with* Avocado *and* Cream Cheese

★ :: **MAKES 4**

I feel okay tweaking this crunchy American classic in the name of health. My take on the BLT is a pita with turkey bacon and fat-free cream cheese instead of mayo. Avocado slices are my nod to sunny California.

8 turkey bacon strips

2 whole wheat pitas, split horizontally

¼ cup fat-free cream cheese

½ Hass avocado, sliced

4 butter lettuce leaves

2 tomatoes, sliced

1 Cook the turkey bacon until crisp over medium heat in a skillet. Drain on paper towels.

2 Spread each pita half gently with 1 tablespoon cream cheese. Top with the bacon, avocado, lettuce, and tomatoes. Roll up and serve.

PER SERVING: 189 calories (36 from fat), 18 g protein, 4 g fat (0 g saturated fat), 23 g carbohydrates, 4 g fiber, 53 mg cholesterol, 277 mg sodium

★

The Hollywood Wrap

Bootylicious

How do Jennifer Lopez, Jessica Biel, and other stars get and keep those shapely derrières?

These pros know how to look good and get the job done. Jennifer has a dance background, and Jessica's built like a gymnast. These are two of the hardest-working women I've ever encountered! Take their lead and get your body moving . . . today!

Take a few moments several times during the day—while chicken breasts are cooking or you're chatting on the phone—and do 20 squats to get those curvaceous cheeks. Stand with your feet shoulder-width apart, cross your arms behind your head, and lower your butt as if you are going to sit in a chair. Rise up slowly, taking care not to lock your knees, and squeeze your glutes as you reach the standing position. Work up to 3 sets of 20 every day.

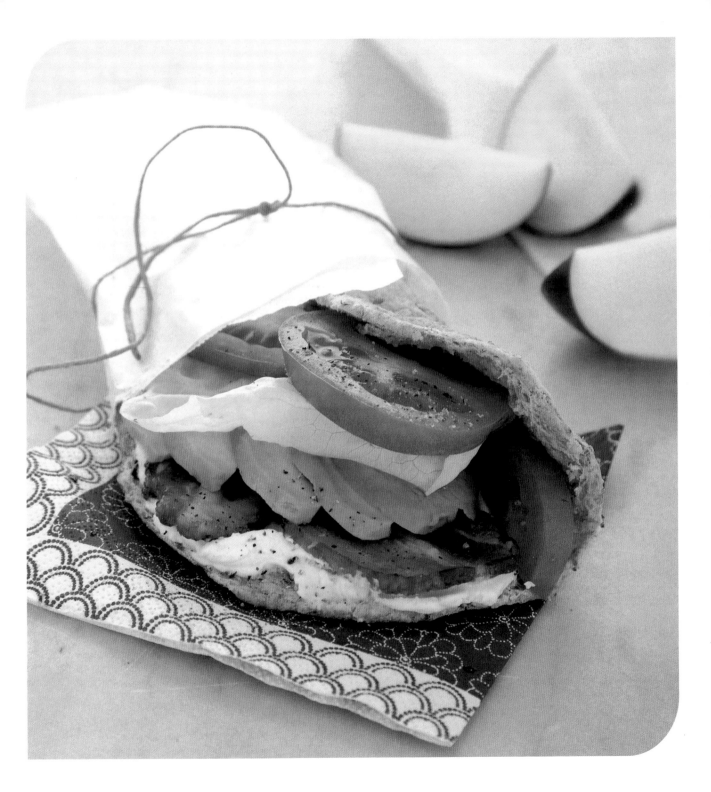

Turkey-Swiss Deli Wraps

A deli sandwich is problematic when made of two slices of white bread piled with salty meat and fatty cheese. You can still enjoy a turkey-and-Swiss 'wich if you follow the Hollywood Wrap rules. Buy low-sodium turkey and low-fat cheese, and instead of mayo, use a fig preserve with less than 5 grams of sugar per teaspoon. Knott's Berry Farm makes Kadota Fig Preserves, which you can buy online at www.smucker.com.

2 tablespoons fig preserves

2 teaspoons extra-virgin olive oil

2 teaspoons red wine vinegar

2 teaspoons chopped kalamata olives

¼ teaspoon Dijon mustard

4 whole wheat tortillas (8-inch)

1 pound sliced low-sodium turkey breast

2 ounces sliced low-fat Swiss cheese

1 large plum tomato, cut crosswise into 8 slices

½ red onion, sliced

1 Whisk together the preserves, oil, vinegar, olives, and mustard in a bowl. Drizzle evenly over the tortillas.

2 Layer the turkey, cheese, tomato, and onion on top. Fold the bottom end of the tortilla up and over the filling, fold in both sides, and continue rolling. Serve.

PER SERVING: 324 calories (52 from fat), 34 g protein, 6 g fat (1 g saturated fat), 40 g carbohydrates, 4 g fiber, 53 mg cholesterol, 1,374 mg sodium

Sloppy Joe Turkey Wraps

This is Halle Berry's fave wrap. For me, it's comfort food that reminds me of family dinners when I was a kid. Ground turkey is bland on its own, but here the onion, red pepper, and garlic powder perk it right up.

1 pound extra-lean ground turkey breast

¼ cup chopped red onion

¼ cup chopped red bell pepper

½ teaspoon garlic powder

¾ cup low-sugar ketchup

1 tablespoon maple syrup

1 teaspoon Dijon mustard

1 teaspoon Truvia

¼ cup fat-free sour cream

4 whole wheat tortillas (8-inch), warmed

1 Heat a skillet over medium-high heat. Coat with cooking spray. Add the turkey and cook, stirring occasionally, until cooked through and browned, 5 to 7 minutes.

2 Stir in the onion and bell pepper and cook for 5 minutes. Stir in the garlic powder, then add the ketchup, maple syrup, mustard, and Truvia and mix thoroughly.

3 Spread 1 tablespoon of sour cream on each tortilla. Divide the turkey mixture evenly among the wraps. Fold the bottom end of the tortilla up and over the filling, fold in both sides, and continue rolling. Serve warm.

PER SERVING: 299 calories (29 from fat), 33 g protein, 3 g fat (0 g saturated fat), 36 g carbohydrates, 3 g fiber, 46 mg cholesterol, 598 mg sodium

Pastrami-Swiss Wraps

★ :: **MAKES 4**

Pastrami and Swiss on rye with Russian dressing is a New York deli classic—and the first thing I want to eat when I step off a plane in the Empire State. This healthy version is packed with lean turkey-pastrami, low-fat Swiss cheese, and a low-fat Russian dressing. I enjoy it frequently without having to travel 3,000 miles!

1/4 cup 0% plain Greek yogurt

2 tablespoons ketchup

1 teaspoon Dijon mustard

2 teaspoons drained capers, finely chopped

4 whole wheat tortillas (8-inch), warmed

1 pound sliced turkey-pastrami

4 slices reduced-fat Swiss cheese

1/4 cup pickled pearl onions, drained and chopped

1 Whisk together the yogurt, ketchup, mustard, and capers in a small bowl.

2 Spread the tortillas with the dressing. Top with the turkey-pastrami, cheese, and onions. Fold the bottom end of the tortilla up and over the filling, fold in both sides, and continue rolling. Serve.

PER SERVING: 351 calories (95 from fat), 34 g protein, 11 g fat (4 g saturated fat), 30 g carbohydrates, 3 g fiber, 90 mg cholesterol, 1,433 mg sodium

Barbecued Turkey Meatball Wraps

★ :: **MAKES 4**

Barbecue sauce adds the kick and oatmeal adds the texture to these low-fat meatballs. Double the recipe and freeze some for yummy wrapping later on.

10 ounces extra-lean ground turkey breast

$\frac{1}{2}$ cup quick-cooking oatmeal

$\frac{1}{4}$ cup + 2 tablespoons Barbecue Sauce (page 97) or Bull's-Eye Barbecue Sauce

$\frac{1}{4}$ cup chopped parsley

$\frac{1}{4}$ cup finely chopped onion

$\frac{1}{4}$ cup crumbled fat-free feta cheese

2 tablespoons low-sodium chicken broth

1 egg white

3 garlic cloves, minced

$\frac{1}{2}$ teaspoon dried oregano

$\frac{1}{8}$ teaspoon freshly ground black pepper

$\frac{1}{8}$ teaspoon grated nutmeg

4 whole wheat tortillas (8-inch), warmed

1 Preheat the oven to 375°F. Coat a non-stick baking sheet with cooking spray.

2 Using your hands, mix together the turkey, oatmeal, $\frac{1}{4}$ cup of the barbecue sauce, the parsley, onion, feta, broth, egg white, garlic, oregano, pepper, and nutmeg in a bowl.

3 Divide the mixture into 8 equal portions and shape each portion into a meatball. Arrange them 2 inches apart on the baking sheet. Drizzle the remaining 2 tablespoons of barbecue sauce over the meatballs.

4 Bake the meatballs for 25 minutes, or until browned. Slice the meatballs in half and divide among the tortillas. Fold the bottom end of the tortilla up and over the filling, fold in both sides, and continue rolling. Cut in half and serve.

PER SERVING: 317 calories (30 from fat), 27 g protein, 3 g fat (0 g saturated fat), 47 g carbohydrates, 5 g fiber, 29 mg cholesterol, 749 mg sodium

Meatball Hero Wraps

Who doesn't love a meatball sub? This one is lean and mean, made with white ground turkey breast instead of ground beef. The marinara sauce is fat free and adds flavor and texture to every bite.

1 pound extra-lean ground turkey breast

½ cup grated reduced-fat Parmesan cheese

¼ cup whole wheat panko bread crumbs

¼ cup chopped parsley

3 eggs whites, lightly beaten

2 tablespoons fat-free milk

1 teaspoon dried oregano

¼ cup Marinara Sauce (page 53)

4 ounces shredded provolone cheese

4 whole wheat tortillas (8-inch)

1 Preheat the oven to 350°F.

2 Using your hands, mix together the turkey, Parmesan, panko, parsley, egg whites, milk, and oregano in a bowl. Divide the turkey mixture into 8 equal portions and shape each portion into a ball. Flatten them slightly with the palm of your hand.

3 Heat an ovenproof skillet over medium-high heat. Coat with cooking spray. Add the meatballs and brown all over for 6 to 8 minutes. Transfer the skillet to the oven and bake the meatballs for an additional 10 minutes.

4 Remove from the oven. Spoon the marinara sauce evenly over the meatballs, sprinkle on the cheese, return to the oven, and cook for 3 minutes, until the cheese melts.

5 Place two meatballs on each tortilla. Top them with some sauce. Fold the bottom end of the tortilla up and over the filling, fold in both sides, and continue rolling. Serve warm.

PER SERVING: 474 calories (98 from fat), 48 g protein, 11 g fat (5 g saturated fat), 44 g carbohydrates, 5 g fiber, 80 mg cholesterol, 1,056 mg sodium

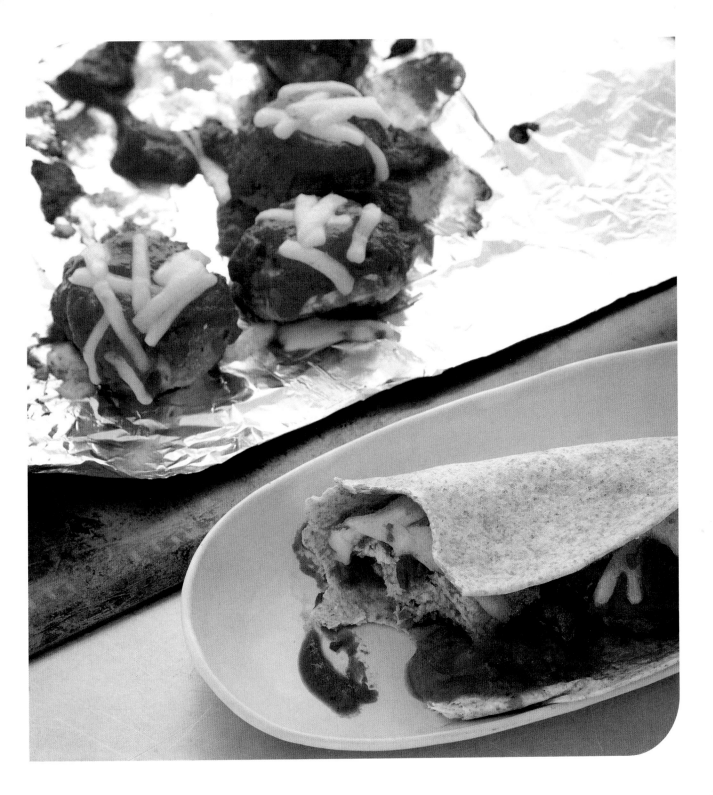

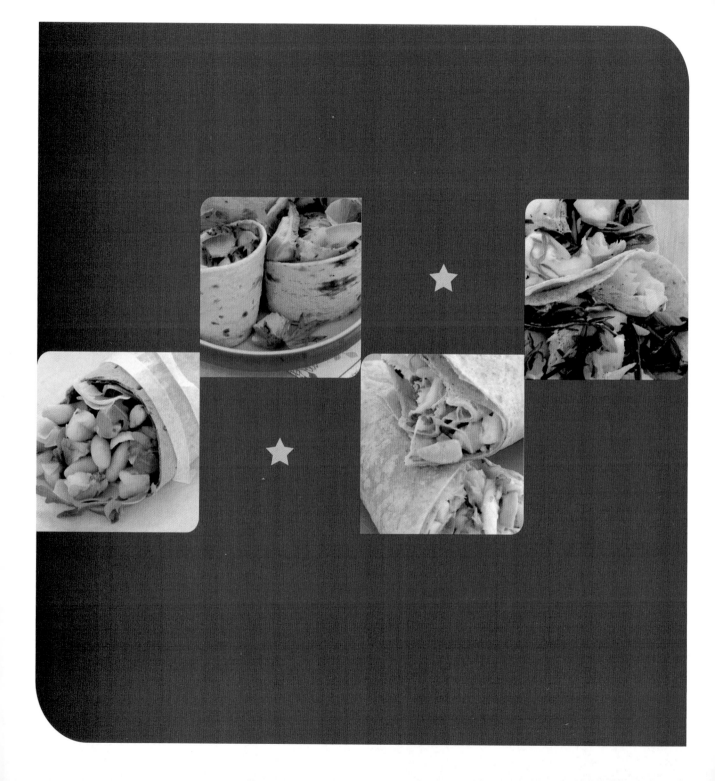

★ Seafood Wraps

Seafood—fish and shellfish—is often overlooked when it comes to making wraps. It's healthy—think omega-3s, which prevent heart disease, help lower blood pressure, and help prevent strokes. It also contains valuable vitamins and minerals. Just as important, seafood tastes great, comes in lots of varieties, is easy to keep on hand, and can be prepared in no time.

Keep a bag or two of frozen shrimp in your freezer. They can be defrosted and cooked up in a flash to make all kinds of substantial wrap fillings. Stock your pantry with canned tuna, sardines, and salmon, too.

You don't have to make big changes to the way you eat to get the great taste and health benefits of seafood. Just eating it twice a week can make a big difference to your health and body. Here are some ways to make upping your fish quotient fun and easy.

Shrimp Cocktail On-the-Go Rolls

★ :: **MAKES 4**

This wrap is a twist on the beloved steak-house starter.

½ **teaspoon fresh lemon juice**

½ **cup ketchup**

1½ **teaspoons prepared horseradish**

1 **pound cooked shrimp, peeled and diced**

4 **iceberg lettuce leaves**

1 Whisk together the lemon juice, ketchup, and horseradish in a bowl.

2 Add the shrimp to the sauce and mix. Fill the lettuce leaves with the shrimp, roll into neat packages, and serve.

PER SERVING: 147 calories (16 from fat), 20 g protein, 2 g fat (0.5 g saturated fat), 9 g carbohydrates, 0 g fiber, 151 mg cholesterol, 614 mg sodium

Look Star-Bright after a Flight

Red carpet premieres all over the world via private Gulfstream jets. Passenger plane press junkets to promote films. Flights from a movie set in Asia to an awards dinner in Hollywood and then back—in less than 48 hours. It all sounds very glamorous, but I've accompanied enough stars on these trips to tell you that celebrities become as jet-lagged, exhausted, and frazzled as the rest of us. No matter what kind of plane you're on, you can't escape time zone changes and the effects of high altitudes on the body which wreak havoc on skin, eyes, and sleep patterns.

Water is extra important during travel. Pack a large, empty water bottle in your purse or carry-on tote. Once you're through security, fill it at the nearest water fountain and drink frequently to stay hydrated.

Avoid drinking alcohol on the plane. I know, you may want to get a jump start on that vacation, but alcohol is dehydrating. It takes 8 ounces of water to metabolize 1 ounce of alcohol. Do the math.

Pack a wrap or two to bring, along with some fresh fruit. If you're prepared, you won't give in to the high-fat, high-sodium snacks and sandwiches offered.

Once you arrive at your destination, eat small meals throughout the day to allow your body to adjust. Keep a snack by your bed. Exercise in the morning to help reset your internal clock.

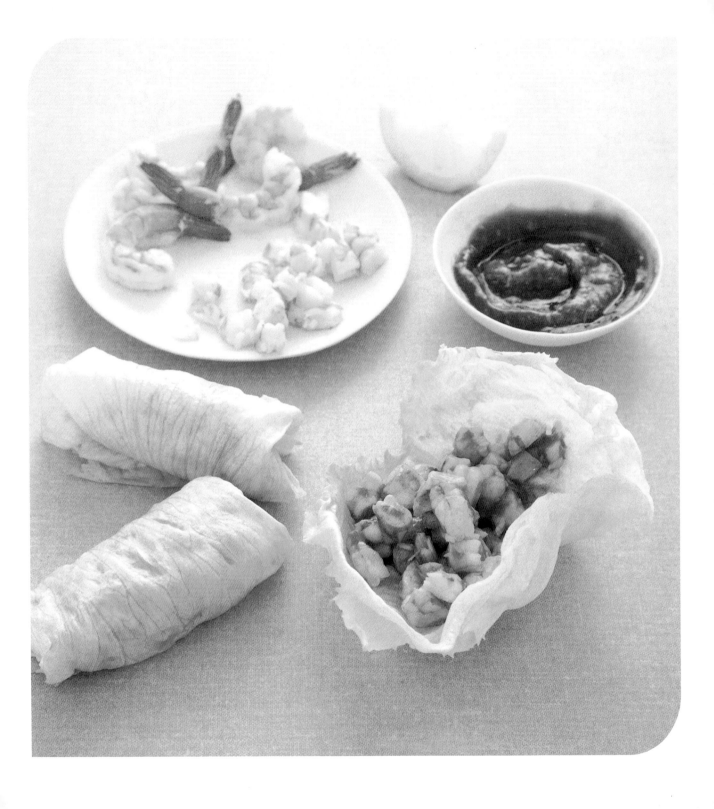

Shrimp-Asparagus Rolls

These shrimpy delights are elegant enough to slice and serve at a cocktail party and casual enough to tuck into a brown bag lunch. Steamed broccoli florets or baby bok choy can replace the asparagus, and if you want to splurge, fresh crabmeat or lobster can stand in for the shrimp.

⅓ cup fat-free, low-sodium chicken broth

3 tablespoons fresh lemon juice

2 tablespoons honey

1 tablespoon low-sodium soy sauce

1 tablespoon grated lemon zest

1 tablespoon grated fresh ginger

1 teaspoon minced garlic

1 teaspoon Sriracha chili sauce

1 teaspoon arrowroot

2 tablespoons extra-virgin olive oil

1 cup asparagus tips (about 2 inches long)

1 pound shrimp, peeled and deveined

¼ cup chopped cilantro

4 garlic-flavored whole wheat tortillas (8-inch)

1 cup cooked brown rice

1 Whisk together the broth, lemon juice, honey, soy sauce, lemon zest, ginger, garlic, and chili sauce in a bowl. Add the arrowroot and whisk to dissolve.

2 Heat a skillet over high heat. When hot, add 1 tablespoon of the oil and the asparagus tips. Stir-fry until crisp-tender, 3 to 5 minutes. Using tongs, remove the asparagus to a bowl.

3 Add the remaining 1 tablespoon oil to the skillet. Add the shrimp and stir-fry until they turn pink, about 3 minutes. Return the asparagus to the pan, add the sauce and cilantro, and toss and stir for 1 minute.

4 Spread one-quarter of the asparagus-shrimp mixture in the middle of each tortilla, leaving a ½-inch border on the sides and bottom. Top each with ¼ cup of brown rice. Fold the bottom end of the tortilla up and over the filling, fold in both sides, and continue rolling. Serve warm.

PER SERVING: 402 calories (95 from fat), 27 g protein, 11 g fat (1 g saturated fat), 51 g carbohydrates, 5 g fiber, 153 mg cholesterol, 650 mg sodium

Lime-Glazed Shrimp Tacos

Fish tacos made their way up through California from Mexico to become a West Coast fave. It wasn't long before someone decided to replace the fish with shrimp—and I became so addicted to the variations that I had to start making my own. Now, my clients are the ones begging for these tacos. The mango chutney you need for the sauce is readily available in jars in supermarkets.

⅓ cup honey-Dijon mustard

¼ cup mango chutney

2 tablespoons fresh lime juice + 1 lime, cut into wedges

1 tablespoon Truvia

1 teaspoon grated lime zest

1 tablespoon canola or olive oil

1 pound large or jumbo shrimp, peeled and deveined

1 large red or green bell pepper, cut into 1-inch pieces

1 cup cooked brown rice

4 whole wheat tortillas (8-inch), warmed

1 Whisk together the mustard, chutney, lime juice, Truvia, and lime zest in a bowl. Set aside.

2 Heat the oil in a skillet over medium-high heat. Add the shrimp and bell pepper, and cook, stirring frequently, until the shrimp turn pink. Stir in half of the mustard-lime sauce and toss to coat.

3 Divide the brown rice among the tortillas, leaving a ½-inch border on the sides and bottom. Top with the shrimp mixture. Drizzle on the remaining sauce. Fold the bottom end of the tortilla up and over the filling, fold in both sides, and continue rolling. Serve with the lime wedges.

PER SERVING: 438 calories (65 from fat), 26 g protein, 7 g fat (1 g saturated fat), 64 g carbohydrates, 5 g fiber, 151 mg cholesterol, 746 mg sodium

Shrimp, Artichoke, *and* White Bean Wraps

★ :: **MAKES 4**

Serve this part-ocean, part-garden mixture nestled in tortillas or on a bed of mixed baby lettuces. Or add some chopped tomatoes and toss with some whole wheat rotini. The options are endless! Use canned or frozen artichokes for convenience.

1 teaspoon + 2 tablespoons extra-virgin olive oil

1 pound large shrimp, peeled, deveined, and chopped

$\frac{1}{2}$ cup canned cannellini beans, rinsed and drained

6 ounces canned artichoke hearts, rinsed and chopped

2 tablespoons fresh lemon juice

Freshly ground black pepper

4 whole wheat tortillas (8-inch), warmed

2 cups arugula

1 Heat 1 teaspoon of the oil in a skillet over medium heat. Add the shrimp and cook until they turn opaque, no more than 3 to 4 minutes. Remove the shrimp to a bowl and let cool.

2 Once the shrimp are at room temperature, add the beans, artichokes, the remaining 2 tablespoons of oil, the lemon juice, and pepper to taste and toss well.

3 Spread one-quarter of the shrimp salad on each tortilla, leaving a $\frac{1}{2}$-inch border on the sides and bottom. Add a handful of arugula to each. Fold the bottom end of the tortilla up and over the filling, fold in both sides, and continue rolling. Serve.

PER SERVING: 357 calories (103 from fat), 28 g protein, 11 g fat (1.5 g saturated fat), 36 g carbohydrates, 5 g fiber, 151 mg cholesterol, 616 mg sodium

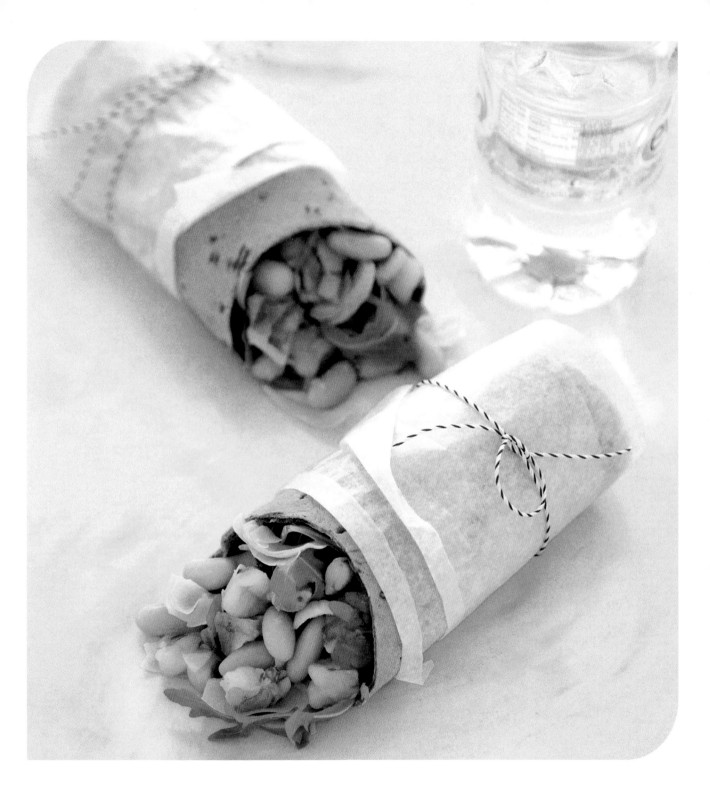

Crab, Shrimp, *and* Avocado Rolls

With a double dose of seafood, these wraps are loaded—and I mean loaded—with protein plus essential fats from the avocado. Serve these as an appetizer at your next bash.

1 can (4.5 ounces) crabmeat or 4½ ounces fresh crabmeat

4 ounces cooked peeled and deveined shrimp, coarsely chopped

¼ cup peeled, diced cucumber

¼ cup diced tomato

Sriracha chili sauce

2 tablespoons fat-free mayonnaise

1 tablespoon fresh lemon juice

1 teaspoon Dijon mustard

¼ teaspoon freshly ground black pepper

1 Hass avocado, diced

¼ cup chopped cilantro

4 spinach-flavored whole wheat tortillas (8-inch), warmed

1 Toss the crab, shrimp, cucumber, tomato, chili sauce to taste, mayonnaise, lemon juice, mustard, and pepper together in a bowl. Cover and refrigerate for 1 hour to blend the flavors.

2 Just before serving, add the avocado and cilantro and mix well.

3 Spread one-quarter of the seafood mixture in the middle of each tortilla, leaving a ½-inch border on the sides and bottom. Fold the bottom end of the tortilla up and over the filling, fold in both sides, and continue rolling. Serve.

PER SERVING: 481 calories (155 from fat), 23 g protein, 17 g fat (2 g saturated fat), 58 g carbohydrates, 6 g fiber, 95 mg cholesterol, 852 mg sodium

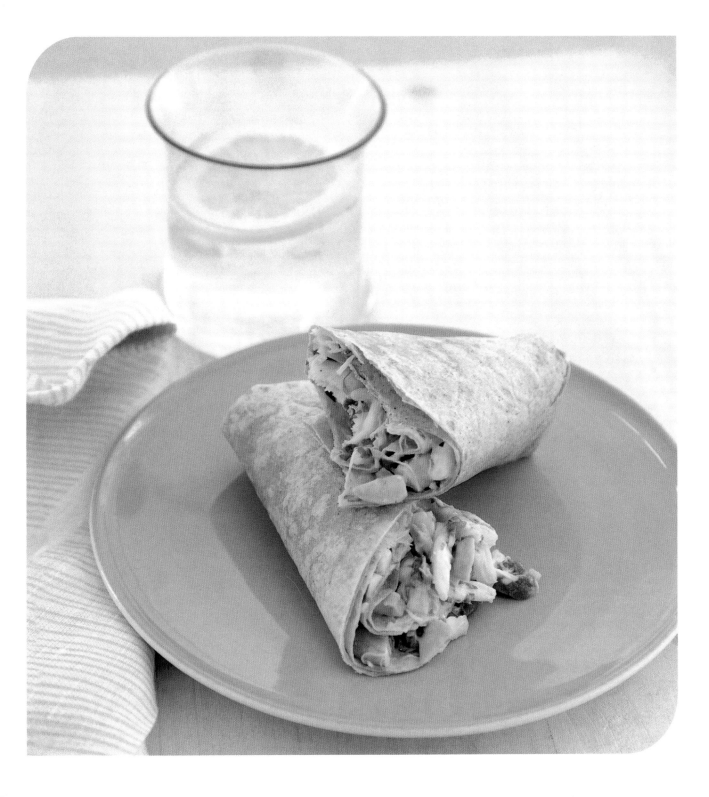

Seafood Salad Wraps

Love seafood salad? Use all scallops or all shrimp for this creamy concoction, or add some lobster meat, depending on your budget and what's available in your market. Another idea might be cooked calamari or steamed mussels. You will have to adjust the recipe according to which seafood you use, as some comes frozen and cooked, and some comes uncooked. Follow the instructions on the package and you should be good to go.

1 tablespoon extra-virgin olive oil

12 ounces bay scallops

2 tablespoons fat-free sour cream

2 tablespoons fat-free mayonnaise

2 tablespoons fresh lime juice

2 tablespoons chopped scallions

½ jalapeño pepper, seeded and minced

12 ounces cooked peeled and deveined shrimp

4 romaine lettuce leaves, center ribs cut out

2 tomatoes, diced

½ Hass avocado, diced

1 Heat the oil in a skillet over medium-high heat. Add the scallops and cook, stirring constantly, for 1½ to 2 minutes. Don't overcook them. Transfer them to a bowl to cool.

2 Combine the sour cream, mayonnaise, lime juice, scallions, and jalapeño. Add the shrimp and scallops and stir gently to coat with the dressing.

3 Divide the seafood salad among the lettuce leaves and top with the tomatoes and avocado. Roll up and serve.

PER SERVING: 343 calories (75 from fat), 34 g protein, 8 g fat (1 g saturated fat), 11 g carbohydrates, 3 g fiber, 195 mg cholesterol, 403 mg sodium

Cod with Brown Rice in Lettuce Leaves

★ :: **MAKES 4**

Nothing like fresh fish for a lean, flavor-blasted meal. Cod is meaty and super satisfying, but if you can't find it, just about any firm white fish such as halibut or haddock works in this Asian-inspired wrap. Serve the fish in lettuce leaves and accompany with a cool seaweed salad.

¾ cup honey

½ cup low-sodium soy sauce

⅓ cup toasted sesame oil

⅓ cup apple cider vinegar

1 teaspoon grated fresh ginger

1 teaspoon freshly ground black pepper

4 cod fillets (6 ounces each)

4 romaine lettuce leaves

1 cup cooked brown rice

1 Mix together the honey, soy sauce, sesame oil, vinegar, ginger, and pepper in a shallow dish. Add the fish and turn to coat with the marinade. Refrigerate the fish for 30 minutes.

2 Preheat the oven to 450°F. Coat an ovenproof baking dish with cooking spray.

3 Remove the fish from the marinade (discard the marinade) and place in a single layer in the baking dish. Bake for 12 to 15 minutes, until cooked through when pierced with a knife. Spoon the fish onto the lettuce leaves, top with some of the rice, roll, and serve.

PER SERVING: 377 calories (90 from fat), 30 g protein, 10 g fat (2 g saturated fat), 39 g carbohydrates, 1 g fiber, 73 mg cholesterol, 631 mg sodium

Ginger Fish Tacos

Put an Asian spin on fish tacos by adding ginger to the cabbage topping. Use any type of white flaky fish. Serve up with a fresh fruit salsa and some black bean dip.

¼ cup fat-free sour cream

2 tablespoons fresh lime juice

2 cups shredded red cabbage

⅓ cup sliced scallions

1 jalapeño pepper, minced

1 teaspoon minced fresh ginger

1 tablespoon olive oil

Freshly ground black pepper

4 white fish fillets (6 ounces each), such as cod, orange roughy, or halibut

4 Mountain Bread corn wraps or corn tortillas

1 Whisk the sour cream and lime juice together in a large bowl. Transfer half of the mixture to a small bowl and set aside.

2 Add the cabbage, scallions, half of the minced jalapeño, and the ginger to the large bowl and mix well.

3 Heat the oil in a large skillet over medium heat. Add the remaining jalapeño and cook for 1 or 2 minutes, until softened.

4 Pepper the fish lightly on both sides and add to the skillet. Cook until golden brown, 4 to 5 minutes, then turn, using a spatula, and cook for 4 to 5 minutes on the other side. Transfer the fish to a cutting board and slice into small strips.

5 Divide the fish and cabbage salad among the wraps. Top with the reserved sour cream mixture, roll up, tucking in the ends, and serve.

PER SERVING: 260 calories (40 from fat), 34 g protein, 5 g fat (1 g saturated fat), 18 g carbohydrates, 2 g fiber, 75 mg cholesterol, 160 mg sodium

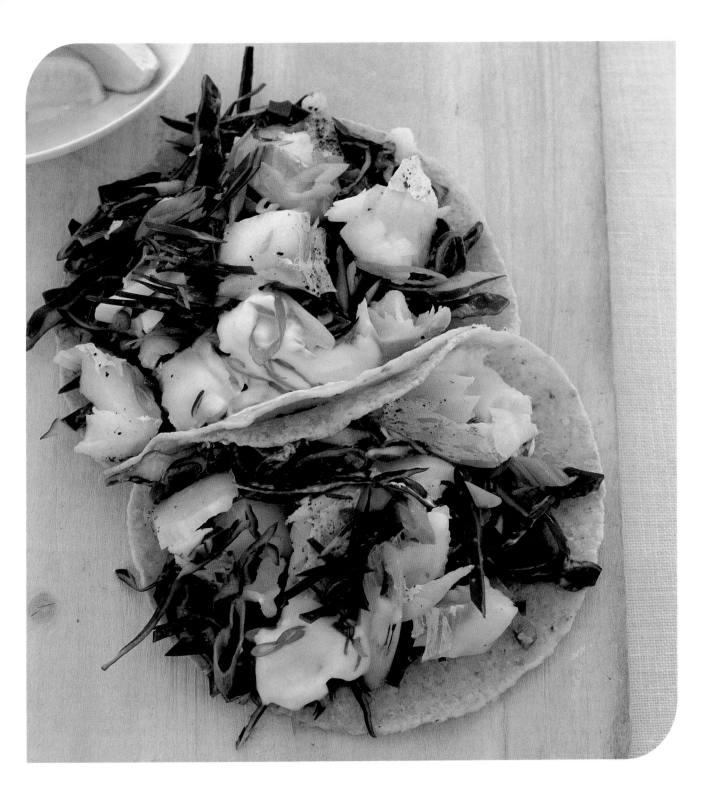

Cajun Salmon *and* Avocado Wraps

Most commercially available Cajun seasoning mixes are loaded with salt, but it's easy to make your own at home. Try this zesty seasoning blend on chicken, steak, shrimp, or tofu. You can cook the fillets and refrigerate for a day or two before wrapping them up.

Cajun Spice Blend

1 teaspoon paprika

1 teaspoon garlic powder

1 teaspoon onion powder

½ teaspoon cayenne pepper

½ teaspoon dried thyme

½ teaspoon freshly ground black pepper

4 salmon fillets (4 ounces each)

4 pieces (8 x 8-inch) whole wheat lavash

2 cups mixed greens

1 Hass avocado, quartered

Lemon-Dill Vinaigrette

3 tablespoons fresh lemon juice

5 teaspoons extra-virgin olive oil

½ teaspoon Dijon mustard

1 teaspoon fresh dill

1 Preheat the oven to 350°F.

2 To make the spice blend: Combine the paprika, garlic powder, onion powder, cayenne, thyme, and black pepper in a small bowl and stir to blend.

3 Using your fingers, pat the spice blend on top of the salmon fillets.

4 Heat a skillet over medium heat. Coat with cooking spray. Add the salmon to the skillet and cook for 3 to 5 minutes on one side. Flip the fillets and cook on the second side for an additional 3 to 5 minutes, or until cooked through. Transfer the salmon to a plate and let rest for 5 to 10 minutes.

5 Flake the salmon and arrange on the lavash. Top with the greens and avocado. To make the vinaigrette: Stir together the lemon juice, oil, mustard, and dill in a small bowl. Drizzle 1 tablespoon over the salmon. Roll up, tucking in the ends, and serve.

PER SERVING: 469 calories (256 from fat), 29 g protein, 28 g fat (5 g saturated fat), 29 g carbohydrates, 7 g fiber, 62 mg cholesterol, 123 mg sodium

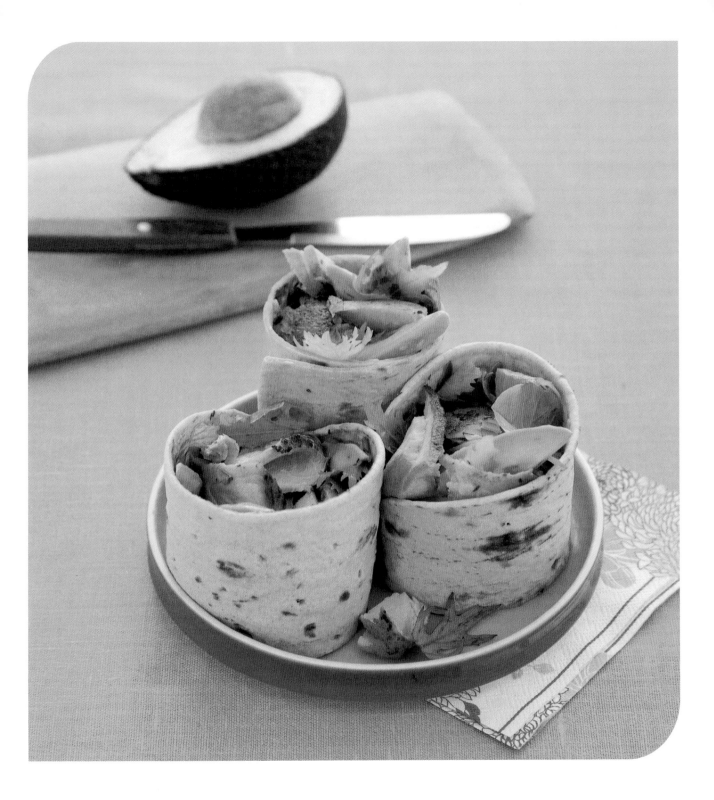

Grilled Salmon Wraps
with Mustard-Dill Sauce

★ :: **MAKES 4**

Mustard-dill sauce is a tasty condiment at many restaurants, but the heavy cream and butter in it are probably not mentioned on the menu. Substitute Greek yogurt and olive oil, and the fat and calorie counts immediately spiral downward. Cook the asparagus to your desired tenderness. I prefer it slightly crunchy.

8 asparagus spears

¾ cup 0% plain Greek yogurt

1 tablespoon honey

1 tablespoon Dijon mustard

1 tablespoon coarse-grained mustard

1 tablespoon extra-virgin olive oil

¼ cup + 2 tablespoons chopped fresh dill

Freshly ground black pepper

4 salmon fillets (6 ounces each)

4 spinach-flavored whole wheat tortillas (8-inch), warmed

1 Bring ½ inch of water to a boil in a skillet. Add the asparagus, cover, reduce the heat, and simmer until the asparagus are cooked but still firm, 1½ to 2 minutes. Using tongs, remove the asparagus to a bowl of ice water to cool. Pat dry and set aside.

2 Preheat the broiler to high or heat the grill.

3 Combine the yogurt, honey, mustards, oil, ¼ cup of the dill, and pepper to taste in a bowl. Mix well. Set aside.

4 Lightly brush a broiler pan or the grill with oil to keep the fish from sticking. Broil or grill the salmon on one side for 3 to 6 minutes. Using a spatula, turn the salmon over and cook for an additional 2 to 3 minutes. Sprinkle the remaining 2 tablespoons dill over the fish.

5 Divide the salmon and asparagus evenly among the tortillas. Top with the sauce. Fold the bottom end of the tortilla up and over the filling, fold in both sides, and continue rolling. Serve.

PER SERVING: 563 calories (251 from fat), 43 g protein, 28 g fat (6 g saturated fat), 34 g carbohydrates, 4 g fiber, 94 mg cholesterol, 477 mg sodium

Crunchie Munchie Tuna Wraps

★ :: **MAKES 4**

Another take on the tuna melt, but this time I've added apple and raisins for sweetness and fiber and walnuts for essential fats.

2 whole wheat pitas, split horizontally

½ cup chopped walnuts

2 cans (5 ounces each) water-packed, no-salt-added solid white tuna, rinsed and drained

1 cup diced apple

½ cup raisins

½ cup fat-free mayonnaise

2 tablespoons Dijon mustard

1 teaspoon curry powder

4 thin slices fat-free Cheddar cheese

1 Preheat the broiler. Arrange the pita rounds on a baking sheet.

2 Place the walnuts in a skillet over medium-high heat. Shake the nuts continuously until they start to turn color, 3 to 5 minutes. Remove immediately from the heat and set aside.

3 Mix together the tuna, apple, raisins, mayonnaise, mustard, and curry powder in a bowl.

4 Spread one-quarter of the tuna mixture on each pita round. Sprinkle with the walnuts and top with a slice of Cheddar cheese.

5 Place the baking sheet under the broiler. Broil for 3 to 5 minutes, until the cheese has melted. Serve hot.

PER SERVING: 341 calories (114 from fat), 24 g protein, 13 g fat (1.5 g saturated fat), 39 g carbohydrates, 8 g fiber, 31 mg cholesterol, 913 mg sodium

Grilled Tuna Rolls

Ask whoever is behind the counter at the fish market to grind up some fresh fish for these to-die-for tuna burgers. If your local market can't do it, then get out the food processor and get grinding on your own. Don't overgrind, though; you want some texture. Mix in wasabi, that sinus-clearing horseradish, to tickle your taste buds.

¼ cup fat-free sour cream

¼ cup fat-free mayonnaise

1 tablespoon fresh lemon juice

1 tablespoon wasabi paste

1 pound tuna steak, finely chopped

2 scallions, thinly sliced

2 tablespoons low-sodium soy sauce

2 teaspoons grated fresh ginger

½ teaspoon freshly ground black pepper

⅓ cup dried whole wheat bread crumbs

2½ tablespoons sesame seeds

4 whole wheat tortillas (8-inch), warmed

1 Whisk together the sour cream, mayonnaise, lemon juice, and wasabi in a bowl. Cover and refrigerate until ready to use.

2 Combine the tuna, scallions, soy sauce, ginger, and pepper in a bowl. Mix well with your hands. Divide the tuna mixture into 4 patties.

3 Mix the bread crumbs and sesame seeds together on a sheet of wax paper. Dredge the tuna burgers in the mixture to coat. Cover and refrigerate for 1 to 3 hours until ready to cook.

4 Heat a skillet or ridged grill pan over high heat. Coat with cooking spray. Add the burgers, reduce the heat to medium, and cook for 5 minutes on each side for a slightly pink interior, or 7 minutes per side for well done.

5 Spread the wasabi dressing on the tortillas. Top each with a tuna burger, fold in half, and serve.

PER SERVING: 357 calories (63 from fat), 35 g protein, 7 g fat (1 g saturated fat), 41 g carbohydrates, 6 g fiber, 54 mg cholesterol, 886 mg sodium

Niçoise Salad Wraps

A *salade Niçoise* is like a French summer on a plate. Here, it's a French summer wrapped up in romaine leaves. You could also use grilled fresh tuna, salmon, or swordfish in place of the canned tuna.

6 ounces small red potatoes

6 ounces green beans

2 tablespoons fat-free mayonnaise

1 tablespoon white wine vinegar

1 teaspoon fresh lemon juice

1 teaspoon Worcestershire sauce

1 teaspoon Dijon mustard

1 tablespoon chopped fresh dill

1 teaspoon minced garlic

6 cups chopped baby greens

12 cherry tomatoes, quartered

$\frac{1}{2}$ small cucumber, sliced

$\frac{1}{4}$ cup chopped black olives

3 cans (5 ounces each) water-packed, no-salt-added solid white tuna, rinsed and drained

4 romaine lettuce leaves, center ribs cut out

1 Put the potatoes in a pot and cover with water. Bring the water to the boil. Reduce the heat and cook for 10 minutes, then add the green beans to the pot. Cook until the potatoes are just tender when pierced with a fork, about 5 minutes longer. Cut the green beans into 1-inch pieces. Set aside.

2 Whisk together the mayonnaise, vinegar, lemon juice, Worcestershire sauce, mustard, dill, and garlic in a large bowl.

3 Add the potatoes, beans, greens, tomatoes, cucumber, olives, and tuna and toss well to combine.

4 Divide among the lettuce leaves, roll, and serve.

PER SERVING: 186 calories (35 from fat), 22 g protein, 4 g fat (1 g saturated fat), 17 g carbohydrates, 5 g fiber, 34 mg cholesterol, 227 mg sodium

Tuna *and* Black Bean Wraps

In Italy, canned tuna and white beans are often combined and served as an antipasto. I head south of the border with this version by using black beans and salsa to dress up the tuna. If you want to stay in Italian mode, combine tuna, cannellini beans, chopped celery, and a bit of olive oil, and tuck it into lavash or put a scoop on a bed of arugula.

3 cans (5 ounces each) water-packed, no-salt-added solid white tuna, rinsed and drained

1/2 cup canned black beans, rinsed and drained

1/4 cup chopped scallions

1/4 cup shredded carrots

3/4 cup Salsa Picante (page 39)

1/2 cup fat-free mayonnaise

2 teaspoons Dijon mustard

4 chipotle-flavored whole wheat tortillas (8-inch), warmed

1 Mix together the tuna, beans, scallions, carrots, salsa, mayonnaise, and mustard in a bowl.

2 Spread one-quarter of the tuna mixture in the middle of each tortilla, leaving a 1/2-inch border on the sides and bottom. Fold the bottom end of the tortilla up and over the filling, fold in both sides, and continue rolling. Serve.

PER SERVING: 275 calories (45 from fat), 25 g protein, 5 g fat (1 g saturated fat), 40 g carbohydrates, 6 g fiber, 36 mg cholesterol, 817 mg sodium

Tuna Melts

The diner classic features more mayo than tuna (a no-no) on white bread (another no-no) that's topped with American cheese (do I need to say it again?) and then broiled until the cheese melts. Here's a healthy, skinny version with less mayo, reduced-fat cheese, and some crisp greens.

2 cans (5 ounces each) water-packed, no-salt-added solid white tuna, rinsed and drained

¼ cup roasted red peppers, cut into strips

⅓ cup fat-free mayonnaise

2 teaspoons Dijon mustard

2 teaspoons drained capers, rinsed

4 pieces (8 x 8-inch) whole wheat lavash

½ cup shredded reduced-fat Swiss cheese

2 cups arugula

1 Preheat the oven to 350°F.

2 Mix together the tuna, peppers, mayonnaise, mustard, and capers in a bowl.

3 Arrange the lavash on a baking sheet. Sprinkle each piece with about 2 tablespoons of cheese.

4 Bake for 2 to 3 minutes, until the cheese melts. Remove from the oven. Let cool 1 or 2 minutes. Top with arugula and tuna mixture. Roll up, tucking in the ends, and serve.

PER SERVING: 240 calories (60 from fat), 21 g protein, 7 g fat (2 g saturated fat), 28 g carbohydrates, 5 g fiber, 30 mg cholesterol, 310 mg sodium

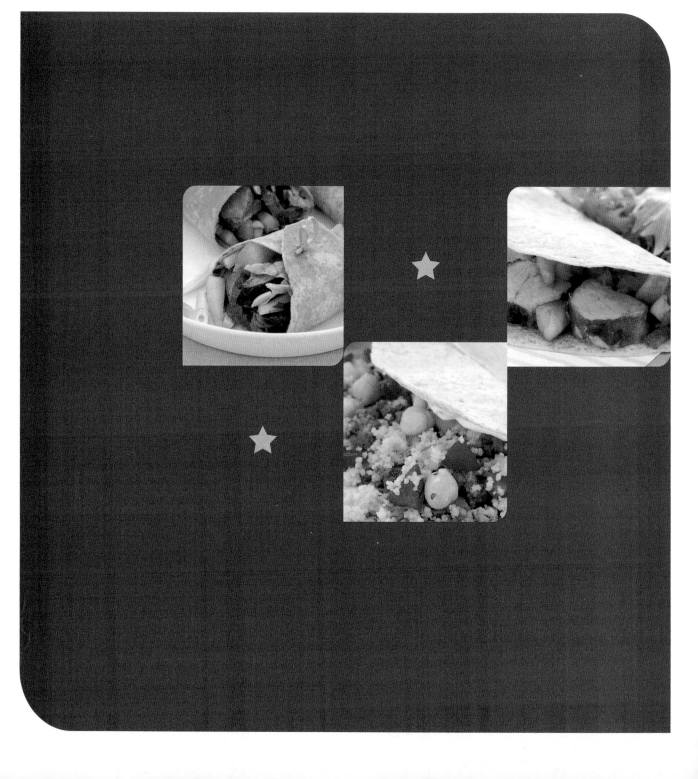

★ Beef, Lamb, and Pork Wraps

Since beef, lamb, and pork come from animals, which means they have saturated fats, they often get a bad rap. You can, however, enjoy them in moderation if you use lean cuts such as filet mignon or sirloin steak, pork tenderloin, and lean ground lamb. Trim off any visible fat before cooking. And whichever you are cooking, keep in mind that no portion should be more than 4 ounces, about the size of a deck of cards.

When buying beef, whenever possible choose meat that comes from grass-fed animals. It is naturally leaner and has more omega-3s and omega-6s than grain-fed beef. (The grain fed to cattle is filled with hormones, to make the animals bigger, and antibiotics, to prevent potential diseases. I don't want any of that stuff in my food, do you?)

And whether you're buying beef, pork, or lamb, it's a good idea to know where your meat comes from and how it was raised and slaughtered. Eatwild.com is a directory that lists more than

1,300 pasture-based farms in the United States and Canada. The farms meet Eatwild's exacting criteria for meat and dairy products—no antibiotics, no hormones, and animals that are humanely treated and not kept in pens. Click on a state, then on a farm in your area, and each farmer describes what animals are raised and how. You can visit many of the farms to pick up beef, lamb, poultry, eggs, and other products, or order by telephone or online for shipment direct to your doorstep. These farms are often owned by generations of the same family; they deserve our support and business even though it's easier to jump in your car and head to the supermarket.

Roast Beef Wraps

Sometimes you've just gotta have some beef. Lean, low-sodium roast beef can be purchased at the supermarket deli counter. Avoid packaged deli meats that are loaded with fillers and sodium. The mayonnaise here is punched up with garlic, a bit of anchovy paste, lemon, and some dill. Use it on other wraps as well or thin it out with a bit of olive oil for a salad dressing.

⅔ cup fat-free mayonnaise

1½ teaspoons anchovy paste

1½ teaspoons fresh lemon juice

2 garlic cloves, minced

½ teaspoon chopped fresh dill

4 pieces (8 x 8-inch) whole wheat lavash bread

1 pound sliced roast beef

4 plum tomatoes, sliced

1 cup chopped spinach

1 Whisk together the mayonnaise, anchovy paste, lemon juice, garlic, and dill in a small bowl. Spread the dressing evenly on the lavash squares.

2 Top each with one-quarter of the roast beef, a few tomato slices, and some spinach. Roll up, tucking in the ends, and serve.

PER SERVING: 280 calories (60 from fat), 27 g protein, 7 g fat (2.5 g saturated fat), 33 g carbohydrates, 6 g fiber, 55 mg cholesterol, 1,380 mg sodium

You Sexy Thing

Rev up your sex life by working out with your significant other. There's nothing hotter than watching your guy or girl pump some iron and do some pushups and seeing those muscles bulge. Trust me, there have been times when I've been mad as heck at my partner, walked into the gym with him, and walked out after a workout needing a shower for two to cool down and cool off. The next thing you know . . .

Mu Shu Beef Wraps

Chinese Mu Shu beef is traditionally high in fat, loaded with salt, and rolled up in pancakes that scream processed white flour. My version uses cabbage leaves as wrappers for fewer carbs, a bit of fiber, and a lot more color. Buy less-sodium soy sauce; it usually has a green label.

4 large red cabbage leaves

1 pound sirloin steak, well trimmed, cut across the grain into 1/2-inch slices

2 teaspoons minced fresh ginger

1 1/2 teaspoons minced garlic

1 cup sliced cremini mushrooms

1/2 cup low-sodium soy sauce

1 tablespoon rice vinegar

1/2 large jalapeño pepper, seeded and minced

2 baby bok choy, halved lengthwise

1 Fill a bowl with ice and water. Bring a large pot of water to a boil. Add the cabbage leaves and cook for 30 seconds to 1 minute, just until the leaves are pliable enough to roll. Using tongs, transfer the leaves to the bowl of ice water to stop the cooking. Dry the cabbage leaves with paper towels and arrange on a work surface.

2 Coat a skillet with cooking spray and heat over high heat. When the skillet is hot, add the steak slices. Cook until medium-rare, about 2 minutes. Using tongs, turn the steak and cook on the other side for an additional 2 minutes. Remove the steak to a plate.

3 Reduce the heat to medium. Add the ginger and garlic and cook for 1 minute. Add the mushrooms, soy sauce, vinegar, and jalapeño and cook until the mushrooms are soft, 5 to 7 minutes.

4 Turn off the heat and stir in the bok choy. The residual heat will warm the bok choy. Stir in the beef slices.

5 Fill each cabbage leaf with one-quarter of the beef mixture, roll up, and serve.

PER SERVING: 190 calories (50 from fat), 28 g protein, 5 g fat (2 g saturated fat), 7 g carbohydrates, 1 g fiber, 55 mg cholesterol, 1,150 mg sodium

Rock Star Arms

Wouldn't you love to have sculpted, yet feminine, arms like Jennifer Lopez and Shakira? Well, here's the routine I used when training those fabulous women.

★ Tricep Kickbacks

With your right knee and left hand on a flat bench to support your upper body, place your left foot on the floor. Grasp a 5-pound dumbbell in your right hand with your palm facing toward your body and your arm bent at a 90-degree angle. Keep your upper arm pressed alongside your body. Extend the weight backward and up moving only from the elbow, until your arm is completely straight and parallel to the floor. Squeeze the tricep and hold for a count of one. Do 3 sets of 12 to 15 reps, alternating arms after each set. As you build your comfort level with this exercise, increase your number of "reps" (repetitions of the exercise) to suit your increased athletic ability. Do not overdo it if you are new to this exercise, or you might pull a muscle.

★ Hammer Curls

Stand with feet shoulder-width apart, keeping knees soft. Hold 5-pound dumbbells in front of your body approximately 4 inches apart with palms facing toward you. Slowly raise the dumbbells toward your upper chest. Hold at the top and contract the bicep muscle for one count. Make sure your elbows are tucked at your side at all times. Slowly lower the dumbbells back to the original start position. Do 15 reps of each move, 3 sets. Increase the weight with each set. Don't hyperextend your elbows as you are lowering the dumbbells by swinging your arms. The benefit of this exercise is that you are creating resistance in your muscles by going *slowly*. Be safe when you are working with weights, even if they are only 5 pounds to start.

So much of having a lean physique depends on having the right muscle-to-fat ratio. What you eat is just as important as how often you work out when it comes to building muscle. Don't let all those gym hours go to waste by eating junk food. Stick with my high-protein Hollywood Wraps to trim your body fat and to these exercises for buff, ripped arms. Then you can wear short sleeves or go sleeveless with no fear of the dreaded "jiggles"!

Asian Steak Salad Wraps

Beef salads are popular throughout much of Southeast Asia, especially Thailand, Cambodia, and Indonesia. Fill tortillas with this sumptuous steak salad or serve by itself—it's definitely meaty enough!

¼ cup Dijon mustard

¼ cup low-sodium teriyaki sauce

1 tablespoon grated fresh ginger

½ teaspoon minced garlic

1 pound flank steak

4 cups chopped mixed salad greens

1 cup chopped yellow or orange bell pepper

2 scallions, thinly sliced

½ cup dry roasted unsalted peanuts

4 garlic-flavored whole wheat tortillas (8-inch)

1 Preheat a grill pan over high heat.

2 Combine the mustard, ½ cup of water, the teriyaki sauce, ginger, and garlic in a small bowl.

3 Grill the steak in the hot pan for 5 to 7 minutes per side, depending on how you like your steak done. Remove the meat to a platter and let rest for 5 minutes. Thinly slice the steak across the grain.

4 Combine the salad greens, bell pepper, scallions, and peanuts in a large bowl and toss to combine. Add the sliced steak and dressing and toss well.

5 Spread one-quarter of the steak salad in the middle of each tortilla, leaving a ½-inch border on the sides and bottom. Fold the bottom end of the tortilla up and over the filling, fold in both sides, and continue rolling. Serve.

PER SERVING: 440 calories (150 from fat), 34 g protein, 17 g fat (3.5 g saturated fat), 38 g carbohydrates, 6 g fiber, 35 mg cholesterol, 790 mg sodium

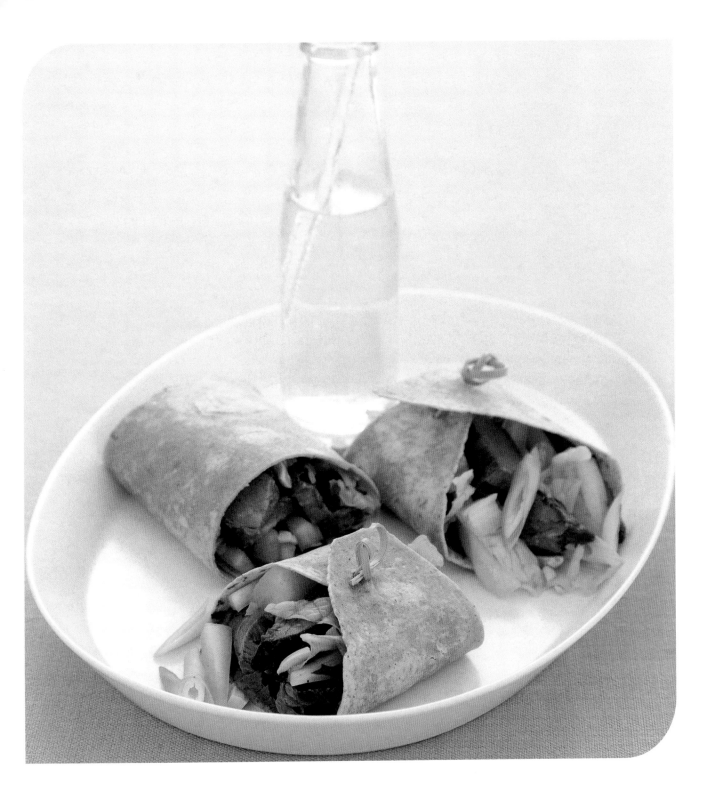

Philly Cheese Steak Wraps

Philly Cheese Steak? Can that really be a Hollywood Wrap? You betcha! My version is mighty lean and clean. Use nonfat or low-fat cheese to reduce fat and calories further.

2 tablespoons fat-free mayonnaise

2 garlic cloves, minced

1 teaspoon fresh lemon juice

2 teaspoons olive oil

1 pound sirloin steak, well trimmed and thinly sliced across the grain

1 large onion, thinly sliced

1 large red bell pepper, sliced

1 green bell pepper, sliced

8 ounces mushrooms, sliced

4 pieces (8 x 8-inch) whole wheat lavash

$\frac{1}{2}$ cup (2 ounces) shredded reduced-fat Swiss cheese

1 Whisk together the mayonnaise, garlic, and lemon juice in a small bowl. Set aside.

2 Preheat the oven to 350°F.

3 Heat the oil in a skillet over medium-high heat. Add the beef, onion, bell peppers, and mushrooms. Cook until the beef is fully cooked and the onions and peppers are softened, 7 to 10 minutes.

4 Arrange the lavash on a baking sheet. Spoon some of the beef mixture on top of each piece, then top with the cheese. Place in the oven for 1 to 2 minutes, just until the cheese melts. Remove from the oven and top with a dollop of the garlic mayo. Roll up, tucking in the ends, and serve.

PER SERVING: 375 calories (115 from fat), 36 g protein, 13 g fat (4 g saturated fat), 34 g carbohydrates, 7 g fiber, 61 mg cholesterol, 181 mg sodium

Steak Wraps *with* Tarragon-Yogurt Sauce

★ :: **MAKES 4**

Get your red meat fix by searing up a piece of beef and wrapping it with tomatoes and this yummy yogurt sauce. If you don't like the taste of tarragon, substitute another fresh herb, like basil or dill.

1 pound sirloin steak, about 1 inch thick, well trimmed

2 tablespoons 0% plain Greek yogurt

½ tablespoon chopped fresh tarragon

1 teaspoon prepared horseradish

2 cups mixed greens

2 plum tomatoes, sliced

4 spinach-flavored whole wheat tortillas (8-inch), warmed

1 Heat a skillet over medium-high heat. Coat with cooking spray. Add the beef and sear on each side for 3 minutes. Continue to cook for 6 to 8 minutes or to your preferred degree of doneness. Remove the steak to a plate to rest for 5 to 10 minutes, then thinly slice across the grain.

2 Whisk together the yogurt, tarragon, and horseradish in a large bowl. Add the sliced meat, greens, and tomatoes and toss well to combine.

3 Arrange one-quarter of the steak mixture in the middle of each tortilla, leaving a ½-inch border on the sides and bottom. Fold the bottom end of the tortilla up and over the filling, fold in both sides, and continue rolling. Serve.

PER SERVING: 300 calories (60 from fat), 30 g protein, 7 g fat (2 g saturated fat), 28 g carbohydrates, 4 g fiber, 55 mg cholesterol, 410 mg sodium

Lamb-Couscous Wraps

This is a great way to use up leftover couscous from last night's meal. Couscous keeps well in the fridge in a covered bowl or plastic bag for up to 3 days, so go ahead and cook up a big batch (no oil or flavorings added, please) to stir into soups, add to salads, or toss with vegetables for a hearty grain salad.

1 teaspoon + 2 tablespoons extra-virgin olive oil

½ large onion, diced

2 teaspoons minced garlic

1 pound ground lamb

½ cup cooked whole wheat couscous

¼ cup chopped cucumber

¼ cup seeded, diced tomatoes

¼ cup canned chickpeas, rinsed and drained

2 tablespoons fresh lemon juice

1 tablespoon chopped parsley

1 tablespoon + 1 teaspoon chopped fresh mint

3 tablespoons 0% plain Greek yogurt

2 whole wheat pitas (8-inch), split horizontally and warmed

1 Heat 1 teaspoon of the oil in a skillet over medium heat. Add the onion and 1 teaspoon of the garlic. Cook, stirring occasionally, until translucent, 3 to 5 minutes. Add the lamb and cook until browned, 5 to 7 minutes.

2 While the lamb is cooking, mix together the couscous, the remaining 2 tablespoons of oil, the cucumber, tomatoes, chickpeas, lemon juice, parsley, and 1 tablespoon of the mint in a large bowl. Set aside.

3 Stir together the yogurt and the remaining 1 teaspoon garlic and 1 teaspoon mint in a bowl.

4 Spread the mint-yogurt sauce on each piece of pita, top with the warm lamb, and finish off with the couscous salad. Roll the pita around the filling and serve.

PER SERVING: 450 calories (280 from fat), 30 g protein, 31 g fat (10 g saturated fat), 12 g carbohydrates, 2 g fiber, 110 mg cholesterol, 110 mg sodium

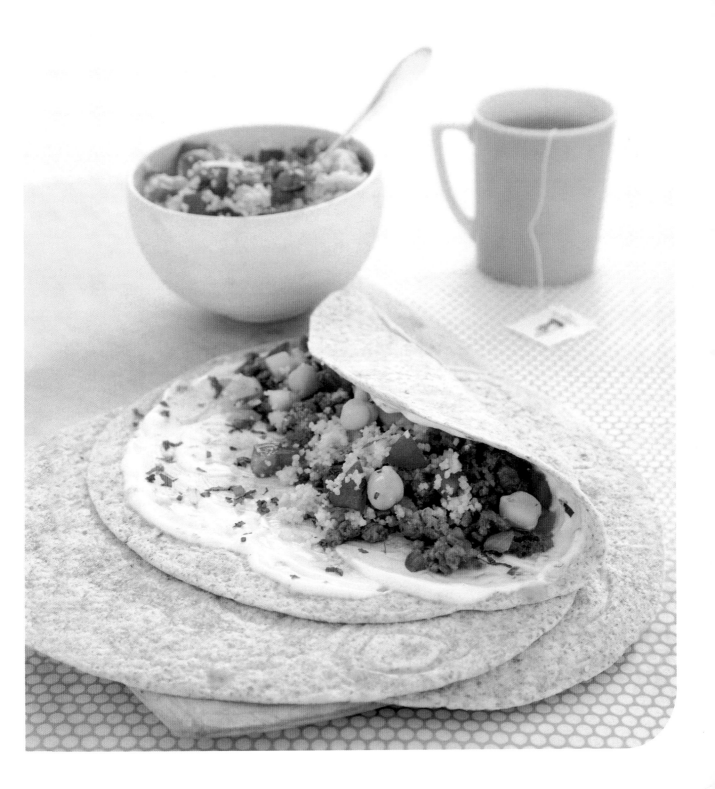

Southern Pork Barbecue Wraps

I was born and raised in the South, where life revolves around who is hosting the next barbecue. Too bad that a lot of southern barbecue faves are loaded with calories, saturated fat, and salt. Well, this homesick southerner decided to create her own healthy version of barbecued pork. With some coleslaw, of course.

1 teaspoon extra-virgin olive oil

1 pound lean ground pork

½ large onion, chopped

¼ cup Barbecue Sauce (page 97) or Bull's-Eye Barbecue Sauce

4 honey-wheat tortillas (8-inch), warmed

Apple Coleslaw

1½ teaspoons honey

1½ teaspoons apple cider vinegar

2½ teaspoons fat-free mayonnaise

½ cup shredded napa cabbage

½ cup shredded red cabbage

½ Granny Smith apple, peeled and shredded

1 Heat a skillet over high heat. Add the oil. When hot, add the pork and onion and cook until the pork is brown, about 10 minutes, stirring to break up the meat. Transfer the pork mixture to a fine-mesh strainer and allow the fat to drain off. Put the pork mixture in a bowl and stir in the barbecue sauce.

2 For the coleslaw, whisk the honey, vinegar, and mayonnaise together in a bowl. Add the cabbages and apples and toss well to combine. (The coleslaw can be made ahead and refrigerated for 1 to 2 days.)

3 Arrange one-quarter of the pork-onion mixture in the middle of each tortilla, leaving a ½-inch border on the sides and bottom. Top with ¼ cup of coleslaw. Fold the bottom end of the tortilla up and over the filling, fold in both sides, and continue rolling. Serve.

PER SERVING: 315 calories (71 from fat), 28 g protein, 8 g fat (2 g saturated fat), 36 g carbohydrates, 3 g fiber, 67 mg cholesterol, 475 mg sodium

Walk Tall

One day a client said, "Working out makes you feel so amazing, you just walk taller, don't you?" She was absolutely right. Exercise is the best self-esteem builder you can have. When you feel better, you look better. And when you look better, you feel better in every way. When you feel great about how you look and feel emotionally, you'll notice that you carry yourself with pride and literally walk a little taller.

To walk even taller, pay attention to your posture. Keep your shoulders back at all times and don't slump. Hold your abs tight; this will force your body to stand tall. Make sure your glutes are tightly tucked, too.

Keeping those glutes tucked in tight as a ballet dancer's creates a good alignment in your back and stretches the length of your spine. My Mom taught me an old beauty school trick: Pretend there's a dime in between your glutes and hold onto that dime all day long. It sounds silly, but trust me, it works!

Hitting a Plateau Is a Message from Your Body

Hitting a plateau means that despite your best efforts—eating well and working out regularly—you're no longer losing pounds. Your body is saying, "I'm bored with our routine, so until you shake it up, I'm not cooperating." What to do?

To keep your body burning fat, building muscle, and losing weight, switch your routine every 4 to 6 weeks. How? Jump on an elliptical trainer or stationary bike instead of running or walking on a treadmill. Try running or jogging outdoors instead of working out indoors. Try machines versus free weights, or the other way around. Take a martial arts or spin class. Use balance boards and medicine balls to challenge your body and your balance. It all pays off. If you *just* diet, you will lose weight for a short amount of time—maybe a month—but exercise is essential to continued and sustained weight loss. If you're not sure what to do, hire a certified personal trainer who can design an exercise regimen specific to you and your body. A qualified trainer will recognize when you've hit a plateau and work with you to revise your program.

Ginger-Peach Pork Wraps

★ :: **MAKES 4**

This is an adaptation of a family favorite. My mother made a variation of this dish when I was a mere slip of a girl, and I've loved it ever since. If fresh peaches are in season, use them. If not, frozen and thawed sliced ones will do. Serve with fresh spinach, sautéed with olive oil and garlic, and a mixed green salad with balsamic vinaigrette.

1½ cups chopped frozen peaches, thawed

½ cup orange all-fruit spread

2 tablespoons low-sodium soy sauce

1½ teaspoons fresh lemon juice

¼ teaspoon ground ginger

¼ teaspoon mustard powder

⅛ teaspoon ground cinnamon

1½ pounds pork tenderloin

4 honey-wheat tortillas (8-inch)

1 Preheat the oven to 350°F.

2 Combine the peaches, fruit spread, soy sauce, lemon juice, ginger, mustard, and cinnamon in a bowl. Mix together well.

3 Place the pork in an ovenproof baking dish and brush all over with the peach glaze. Roast until an instant-read thermometer inserted into the pork reads 160°F, about 1 hour. When done, allow the pork to cool, then slice.

4 Arrange one-quarter of the pork slices in the middle of each tortilla, leaving a ½-inch border on the sides and bottom. Fold the bottom end of the tortilla up and over the filling, fold in both sides, and continue rolling. Serve.

PER SERVING: 430 calories (80 from fat), 39 g protein, 9 g fat (2 g saturated fat), 50 g carbohydrates, 3 g fiber, 110 mg cholesterol, 490 mg sodium

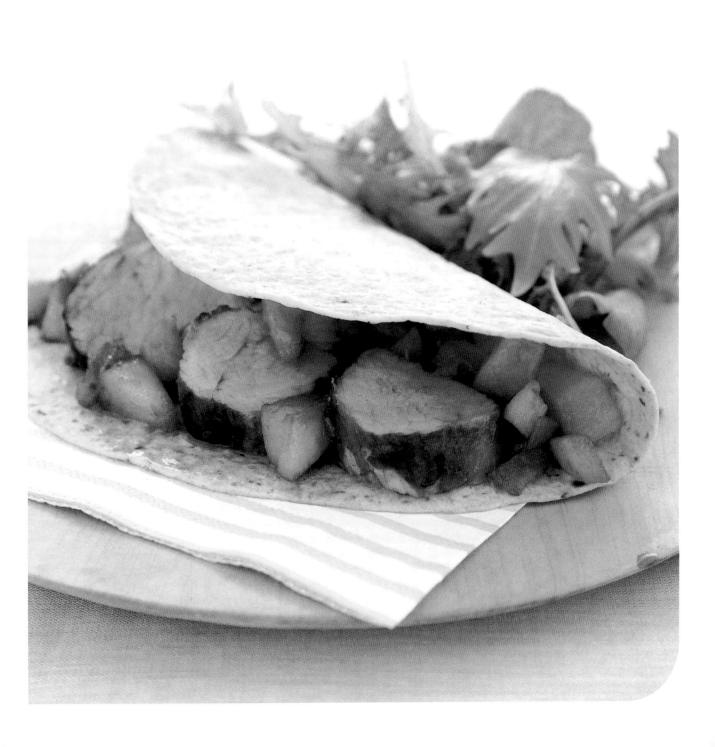

Asian Pork Fried Rice Wraps

Pork tenderloin is a super lean and flavorful cut of meat, often used in Asian cooking. Like American ketchup, Chinese hoisin is a sweet sauce used as a condiment and a cooking ingredient. Look for a brand that's low in sodium. And I don't have to tell you twice to use brown rice instead of white! Serve with some steamed broccoli or bok choy.

1 teaspoon extra-virgin olive oil

1 pound pork tenderloin, cut crosswise into ¹/₂-inch-thick slices

¹/₂ large onion, chopped

2 teaspoons minced garlic

1 teaspoon minced fresh ginger

¹/₂ cup shredded carrots

¹/₂ cup frozen peas, thawed

1 cup cooked brown rice

1 tablespoon low-sodium soy sauce

1 tablespoon low-sodium hoisin sauce

4 whole wheat tortillas (8-inch)

1 Heat a skillet over high heat. Add the oil and when hot, add the pork. Reduce the heat to medium-high and stir-fry until the pork turns brown, 3 to 5 minutes.

2 Add the onion and cook until translucent, 3 to 5 minutes. Stir in the garlic, ginger, carrots, and peas. Add the rice, soy sauce, and hoisin sauce. Mix together well.

3 Spread one-quarter of the fried rice mixture in the middle of each tortilla, leaving a ¹/₂-inch border on the sides and bottom. Fold the bottom end of the tortilla up and over the filling, fold in both sides, and continue rolling. Serve warm.

PER SERVING: 360 calories (50 from fat), 30 g protein, 6 g fat (1 g saturated fat), 44 g carbohydrates, 5 g fiber, 75 mg cholesterol, 600 mg sodium

Acknowledgments

My passion for food long predates my career in health and fitness, and was cultivated far from the limelight—mostly in the kitchens of famous Beverly Hills restaurants, like La Scala, where I waited tables. Over the years many individuals, friends, family members, and strangers have helped me create unique and stylish recipes, many of which are collected here.

Creating this book also relied on the collaboration of many. Thank you to my editor, Pam Krauss, and the entire Rodale team for helping to bring my work to life on the page. Thank you to Kara Plikaitis, photographer Heather Weston, and food and prop stylist Deborah Williams for the beautiful food photography and to my cowriter, Harriet Bell, for always believing in me and supporting me throughout this process. Thank you to my agent, Celeste Fine, at Folio Literary Management, for her expertise and passion. Thank you to Allison Elliot and Susan Brightbill for their loyalty and friendship.

And special thank-yous to Halle Berry, who encouraged me to write this book; Julia Roberts, who gave me my start in this industry; Kevin Costner, who helped me with my first end credit; Jennifer Lopez, who supported me with her worldly advice; and Elliot Gould and Jennifer Love Hewitt for loving my wraps and training style. I am also extremely grateful for Steven Spielberg's constant support. I have stood in my kitchen most Sundays for years preparing his foods. I have shipped my meatballs to him on location, and he is a huge fan of my turkey chili—I'm always careful to portion it correctly, otherwise he'd eat it all in one sitting!

For always being the consummate cheerleaders and supporting my dreams and visions, I would also like to acknowledge David Sobel Photography, Herman Valentine, Dennis Tito, Cindy Cooper, Colin Brown, Danielle Clark Donald, Molly Berke, Elizabeth Thompson, Lenora Marouani and Adnen Marouani, Dawn Steel, Ann Sweeney, John Riley, Kirk Kinzett, Doug Blasdell, Cindy Johnson, Brent Martin, Paul Bland, Steve Bessen, David and Rosanne Fabrizio, Michael Monterosa, Susan Becker, Carol Hannah, Bobbe Bramson, Dr. David Heber, David Allen, Susan Bowerman, Maurice Tuchman, Ted a.k.a. Teddy Sowell, Angel Banos, Sandy Hale, Mary Cunningham, Carroll Thomas, Karen Tencer, John Riley, Steve Sandler, Dr. Alan Rosenbach, Jeff Briggs at Golden Farms, Jesse Heer, Jeff Palmatier a.k.a. Big Bull, Marc Ippolito, Terri Groves,

Sheila Matian, Stacey Bender at BHG PR, French's mustard, Tumaro's Tortillas, Roy Grillo, Carol Oppenheimer, Richard D'Alessandro, Danny Lima and Jon Eric, and Kristin, Margie, and Millie Strom.

And finally, my eternal gratitude to my sisters, Catherine and Sue, who are my constant rocks and best friends, and to my granny and grandmother, whose culinary passion set the groundwork for my career. I also want to thank my dad for showing me the way of the world and exposing me to the big city, jazz, and a love of food. I am also extremely grateful for the patience of my amazing son as I pursued my career and for my granddaughter Kali, who is my kitchen-counter buddy. In true Hollywood spirit, I must include special thanks to my three amazing dogs: Barry, Sammy, and Daisy.

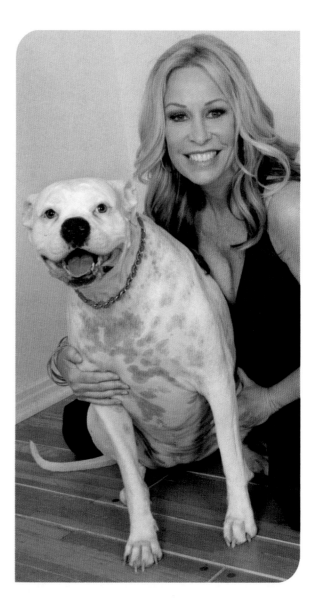

Index

Underscored page references indicate boxed text. **Boldfaced** page references indicate photographs.